S0-BXE-393

[World Health Organization]

THE SI
FOR THE HEALTH
PROFESSIONS

Prepared at the request of the
Thirtieth World Health Assembly

*RB40
W794
1977*

WORLD HEALTH ORGANIZATION
GENEVA
1977

337718

Contents

Acknowledgements

Since no account of the SI could be truly authoritative, as called for by the World Health Assembly in resolution WHA30.39, without the approval of the intergovernmental body that is responsible for it, the description of the SI in this book has been approved by the **Bureau international des Poids et mesures (BIPM).** A debt of gratitude is owed to Dr. J. Terrien, Director of the BIPM, for his many helpful comments on the draft manuscript, all of which have been taken into account in the preparation of the present text.

Official recommendations on the practical application of the SI in different medical specialties, especially clinical chemistry, hematology, and radiology, are primarily a matter for the appropriate international nongovernmental body. The manuscript was consequently submitted to the organizations listed below. These bodies, and particularly the individuals mentioned, gave unsparingly of their time to review, discuss, and comment on the manuscript. (However, they bear no responsibility for the accuracy of the numerical values in the tables and lists of conversion factors in Parts 4 and 5.)

International Commission on Radiation Units and Measurements

K. Lidén, *Scientific Secretary* (Sweden); H.O. Wyckoff, *Chairman* (USA)

International Committee for Standardization in Hematology

O.W. van Assendelft (USA); F.J. Eilers (USA); P. Helleman (Netherlands); J. Koepke (USA); S.M. Lewis, *Executive Secretary* (United Kingdom); J. Spaander, *Chairman* (Netherlands); C. Sultan (France)

International Federation of Clinical Chemistry

J. Bierens de Haan (Switzerland); P.M.G. Broughton, *Secretary* (United Kingdom); H. Büttner (Federal Republic of Germany); R. Dybkær, *Vice-President* (Denmark); R.G. Edwards (Australia); J. Frei, *President* (Switzerland); R. Gräsbeck (Finland); A.H. Holtz (Netherlands); A.B. Kallner (Sweden); J.G. Lines (United Kingdom); P. Lous (Denmark); M. Roth (Switzerland); M. Rubin (USA); N.-E. Saris (Finland).

International Union of Pure and Applied Chemistry, Commission on Quantities and Units in Clinical Chemistry & IFCC Expert Panel on Quantities and Units

B.H. Armbrecht (USA); R. Dybkær (Denmark); R. Herrmann (Federal Republic of Germany); K. Jørgensen (Denmark); P. Métais (France); C. Onkelinx (USA); J. C. Rigg (Netherlands); O. Siggaard-Andersen (Denmark); B. F. Visser (Netherlands); R. Zender, *Chairman* (Switzerland)

To all of these, whose careful review of the manuscript, suggestions, and approval of the revised version have rendered this book a truly international cooperative effort, and to the **International Union of Nutritional Sciences** (B. Isaksson, Secretary General, who reviewed the section on the joule in nutrition), the World Health Organization extends its sincere thanks.

Introduction

The use in medicine of the Système international d'Unités (SI) developed by the Conférence générale des Poids et Mesures was endorsed by the Thirtieth World Health Assembly in May 1977 (the full text of resolution WHA30.39 is reproduced on the inside of the front cover). The resolution also called for the World Health Organization to prepare "a succinct, simple, and authoritative account of the SI" for use in the health professions.

This is that account. The main text is divided into 5 parts. The first part is a description of the SI covering the entire system, and not merely those units that are of concern to the health professions, while the second deals with the practical application of SI units in general medical practice and certain medical specialties. The third part, which covers standardization of laboratory reporting, is not part of the SI itself, but summarizes recommendations that have been made for implementing it, principally in clinical chemistry. Part 4 consists of tables of equivalent values in traditional units and SI units for the more important tests, and Part 5 lists conversion factors. The book is designed for all members of the medical and allied professions—physicians in general practice, specialists, nurses, laboratory technologists, and pharmacists, to name but a few—as well as for students in training for any of these professions. However, to avoid undue complexity some of the more limited applications of the SI in medical research have not been included.

The book is a factual description of the SI and of the recommendations that have been made for implementing it. It does not treat the issue of whether or not the change to SI units should be made: the factors involved in that issue have been discussed at length in the literature and were taken fully into consideration by the delegates to the Thirtieth World Health Assembly when they unanimously endorsed the use of the SI. Nor does the book give recommendations on how to make the change to SI units; guidelines on this subject will be published separately.

It is hoped that this authoritative description of the SI, approved by the principal international organizations that are involved, will simplify the transition to the new system and thus help to implement a truly international language of measurement, breaking down barriers to the exchange of health information throughout the world.

Abbreviations

The following abbreviations for the names of organizations are used in this publication:

BIPM   Bureau international des Poids et Mesures
CGPM   Conférence générale des Poids et Mesures
CIPM   Comité international des Poids et Mesures
ICRU   International Commission on Radiation Units and Measurements
ICSH   International Committee for Standardization in Hematology
IFCC   International Federation of Clinical Chemistry
IUB   International Union of Biochemistry
IUPAC   International Union of Pure and Applied Chemistry

Decimal marker

Throughout the tables, the comma is used as the decimal marker ("decimal point"). This makes it possible to use the same tables in versions of the booklet in languages other than English, avoiding costly resetting of the type and thus greatly reducing both the cost of the booklet and the possibility of error. (As noted in the text, many international organizations have indicated a preference for the comma.)

1. What is the SI?

The SI is the culmination of over a century of international effort to develop a universally acceptable system of units of measurement. The great expansion in world trade and exchange of scientific information following the Second World War gave added impetus to the development of such a system, and in 1954 the units that were to form its basis were adopted by the intergovernmental Conférence générale des Poids et Mesures[1] (CGPM). In 1960 (and subsequently) the CGPM expanded the system, and adopted the name Système international d'Unités (International System of Units) and the international abbreviation SI. The SI is essentially an expanded version of the "metric system" that has been in use since 1901.[2]

Structure of the SI

The SI comprises units of three types: base units, derived units, and supplementary units. It also includes a series of prefixes by means of which decimal multiples and submultiples of units can be formed.

Base units

Seven units have been selected to serve as the basis of the system. These *SI base units,*[3] as they are called, are listed in Table 1, together with their symbols and the quantities[4] they measure.

---

[1] The Conférence générale des Poids et Mesures (which now meets every four years), its executive committee (Comité international des Poids et Mesures, CIPM), and its permanent office and laboratory (Bureau international des Poids et Mesures, BIPM, at Sèvres, near Paris, France) are three organs of the Convention du Mètre (Metre Convention). In addition, there are seven "consultative committees", including the Comité consultatif des Unités, which act as advisory bodies to the CIPM. This intergovernmental organization uses French as its only official language, and it is for this reason that the French names are used in this publication. It should be noted that even if the names are translated into other languages, the abbreviations CGPM, CIPM, and BIPM do not change.

[2] A brief explanation of the relationship between the SI and previously used systems of measurement is given in Appendix 1.

[3] The base units have sometimes been referred to in the literature as the "basic" units or the "fundamental" units of the SI. This is misleading, since they are not to be regarded as any more "basic" or "fundamental" than any other units in the system. They simply happen to have been selected as the units on which the system is based.

[4] The English word *quantity* has two equally correct meanings: the everyday meaning "amount", and the more technical meaning "a measurable physical property" (for example, length, height, speed, temperature, and volume are quantities). When the scientist uses the word, he does so with the latter meaning, and it is with this meaning that it is used in this publication.

Table 1. SI base units

Quantity	Name of unit	Symbol for unit
length	metre	m
mass	kilogram	kg
time	second	s
electric current	ampere	A
thermodynamic temperature[a]	kelvin	K
luminous intensity	candela	cd
amount of substance	mole	mol

[a]The thermodynamic temperature scale is based on the relationship between heat and mechanical work, and is independent of the properties of any particular working substance, such as alcohol or mercury. It should be noted that the unit of measurement is "kelvin", not "degree kelvin", and that its symbol is K, not °K.

The base units are defined very precisely, and the constant progress of science makes it necessary to redefine them, from time to time, even more precisely. The definitions are given in Appendix 2, where it is no doubt the definition of the mole that will primarily interest members of the health professions.

Derived units

By multiplying a base unit by itself, or by combining two or more base units by simple multiplication or division, it is possible to form a large group of units known as *SI derived units.* Thus, to take two simple examples, the derived unit of volume is metre cubed, or cubic metre; and the derived unit of speed is metre divided by second, or metre per second. Examples of a few simple derived units are given in Table 2.

Table 2. Some SI derived units

Quantity	Name of derived unit	Symbol for unit
area	square metre	m^2
volume	cubic metre	m^3
speed	metre per second	m/s (or $m \cdot s^{-1}$)
acceleration	metre per second squared	m/s^2 (or $m \cdot s^{-2}$)
substance concentration	mole per cubic metre	mol/m^3 (or $mol \cdot m^{-3}$)

There are a number of rules that must be followed in writing symbols for units. In addition, many readers may be unfamiliar with the use of exponents as listed in the last column of Table 2. The following explanation may be helpful.

Exponents. The use of m² and m³ to mean "m squared" and "m cubed" (or "square m" and "cubic m") respectively is familiar to everyone. Exponents with a minus sign, however, may seem rather forbidding to some readers. In reality there is nothing mysterious about the minus sign: it merely indicates a reciprocal. Thus s^{-1} means the reciprocal of s, or $1/s$; s^{-2} means the reciprocal of s^2, or $1/s^2$, and so on.

Multiplication. Multiplication may be indicated in any of three ways: by a "dot on the line", by a "raised dot", or by a *small* space between two symbols. Thus the symbol for metre second may be written m.s, m · s, or m s. The use of the raised dot is preferred.

Division. Division may be indicated by a solidus (stroke), by a horizontal line, or by negative exponents, as explained above. Thus the symbol for metre divided by second (metre per second) may be written $\frac{m}{s}$, m/s, or m · s^{-1} (or m.s^{-1} or m s^{-1}); mole per cubic metre may be written mol/m³ or mol · m^{-3}, and so forth.

Complex symbols. Great care must be used in writing symbols for complex units. Too often one sees in the literature symbols such as mg/kg/day ("milligram per kilogram of body weight per day"), which is incorrect mathematically since there is no indication of what the denominator is. *No more than one solidus (stroke) should ever be used in the symbol for a unit* unless ambiguity is removed by the use of parentheses. The symbol mentioned above is ambiguous because it could mean either mg/(kg/day) or (mg/kg)/day. In fact, it is the latter that is intended, and it can be seen that the parentheses in (mg/kg)/day remove the ambiguity. However, it would be even better to write mg · kg^{-1} · d^{-1} (d is the international symbol for "day"). In general, the use of negative exponents is preferable in all complex symbols.

The combination of base units to form derived units illustrates one of the main advantages of the SI. Within the system, there is not a single conversion factor to be memorized: the formation of the derived units does not involve any mathematical factor other than 1 (unity). Such a system of units is said to be *coherent.*

A number of SI derived units have been given special names, most of which are the names (or are derived from the names) of scientists who made an outstanding contribution to the field of study concerned. The reason for assigning special names to such units can be illustrated by an example. The SI unit of force is defined as that force which gives, to a mass of 1 unit (1 kg), an acceleration of 1 unit (1 m/s², which means that the speed of the mass increases each second by 1 m/s). The unit of force is therefore kilogram times metre, divided by second squared, (kg · m)/s² or kg · m · s^{-2}. It would, however, be extremely inconvenient to have to use such a cumbersome name and symbol, and for this reason the SI unit of force has been given the simple name newton (symbol: N).

Another example, of great importance in medicine, is pressure. Pressure is the action of force on an area. The SI unit of pressure is therefore defined as a force of 1 unit acting on an area of 1 unit—that is, newton per square metre (N/m²). This in turn has been given the special name pascal (symbol: Pa), which is much simpler to use. (Since the newton is kg · m · s^{-2}, the pascal is, in terms of base units, that factor divided by square metre, or $kg \cdot m \cdot s^{-2} \cdot m^{-2}$, which reduces to $kg \cdot m^{-1} \cdot s^{-2}$.)

The expression of derived units in terms of base units has been explained in some detail because it is important to understand how the SI is constructed. Although the expression of derived units in terms of base units will sometimes be of importance in medical research, this will usually not be the case in general medical practice. For pressure, for example, it will usually be sufficient to remember pascal as the name of the SI unit.

The eighteen SI derived units that have been given special names are listed in Table 3. Only three of these units—the pascal, the joule, and the degree Celsius—are likely to be of any concern in general medical practice, and for this reason their names are printed in bold-face type. (Most of the other units, however, will be of concern to one or another of the medical specialties.)

Table 3. SI derived units with special names

Quantity	Name of unit	Symbol for unit	Derivation of unit[a]
frequency	hertz	Hz	s^{-1}
force	newton	N	$m \cdot kg \cdot s^{-2}$
pressure	**pascal**	Pa	N/m^2
work; energy; quantity of heat	**joule**	J	$N \cdot m$
power; radiant flux	watt	W	J/s
electric charge; quantity of electricity	coulomb	C	$A \cdot s$
electric potential; potential difference	volt	V	W/A
capacitance	farad	F	C/V
(electric) resistance	ohm	Ω	V/A
conductance	siemens	S	A/V
magnetic flux	weber	Wb	$V \cdot s$
magnetic flux density	tesla	T	Wb/m^2
inductance	henry	H	Wb/A
luminous flux	lumen	lm	$cd \cdot sr$
illuminance	lux	lx	$m^{-2} \cdot cd \cdot sr$
Celsius temperature	**degree Celsius**	°C	K
absorbed dose; absorbed dose index; kerma; specific energy imparted (radiation)	gray	Gy	J/kg
activity (of a radionuclide)	becquerel	Bq	s^{-1}

[a] With the exception of those units that can be expressed only in terms of base units, the derived units are expressed, in this column, in terms of other derived units. (These units can, of course, be expressed in terms of base units; thus, the expression for the newton can be substituted for N in the expression $N \cdot m$ for the joule, giving $m^2 \cdot kg \cdot s^{-2}$ as the expression of the joule in base units, and so on down the list.) It will be noticed that two units in this table—the lumen and the lux—are expressed in terms of a unit (steradian) whose symbol is sr (not a base unit); this is explained in the next section.

With one exception, the *symbols* for units consist of either one or two letters, always in roman (upright) type: they are always written in lower-case letters unless the name of the unit is derived from a proper name. In that case the symbol is either a single capital letter or two letters of which only the first is a capital. However, the *names* of SI units are never written with an initial capital letter, even when they are proper names (thus, pascal, not Pascal).

Supplementary units

The supplementary units occupy a somewhat anomalous position in that the CGPM has not decided whether they are to be regarded as base units or derived units. There are only two such units: the unit of plane angle, the radian (symbol: rad), and the unit of solid angle, the steradian (symbol: sr). Just like the base units, the supplementary units can be used to form derived units (see, for example, the lumen and the lux in Table 3). However, neither of them is of concern in general medical practice.

SI prefixes

For many purposes the SI base units and SI derived units are inconveniently large or small (it would, for example, be inconvenient to use the cubic metre for the volume of blood in the human body). To overcome this difficulty, the SI incorporates a series of *SI prefixes,* by means of which it is possible to form decimal multiples and submultiples of SI units. There are sixteen such prefixes, and they are listed in Table 4.

Table 4. SI prefixes

Factor	Prefix	Symbol for prefix	Factor	Prefix	Symbol for prefix
10^{18}	exa	E	10^{-1}	deci	d
10^{15}	peta	P	10^{-2}	centi	c
10^{12}	tera	T	10^{-3}	milli	m
10^{9}	giga	G	10^{-6}	micro	µ
10^{6}	mega	M	10^{-9}	nano	n
10^{3}	kilo	k	10^{-12}	pico	p
10^{2}	hecto	h	10^{-15}	femto	f
10^{1}	deka (US) deca (UK)	da	10^{-18}	atto	a

The four prefixes printed in "boxes" do not conform to the pattern of the others—that is, they are not obtained by successive multiplications by 10^3 or 10^{-3}, and there is a tendency to avoid them in scientific usage.

When the SI prefixes are used, they are joined directly to the names of units, without punctuation of any kind (thus, kiloohm, not kilo-ohm; megaampere, not mega-ampere). The same is true of the prefix symbols, which are joined to unit symbols without intervening space or punctuation (for example: kPa, kilopascal; mlx, millilux).

An SI prefix joined to a unit multiplies that unit by the factor listed in Table 4. Thus the gigajoule, GJ, is equal to 10^9 J (10^9 joules); the kilopascal, kPa, is 10^3 Pa (1 000 pascals); the millimetre, mm, is 10^{-3} m (0,001 metre); and the nanomole, nmol, is 10^{-9} mol (10^{-9} mole).

The use of exponents above is similar to the usage described previously. Thus multiplication by 10^3 means multiplication by 10 x 10 x 10, i.e., by 1 000; multiplication by 10^{-3} means division by 1 000, and so on.

When the symbol for a multiple or submultiple of a unit includes an exponent, the latter applies to both the unit symbol and the prefix symbol. For example, in the symbol for cubic kilometre, km^3, the cube applies both to "kilo" and to "metre"; thus $1\ km^3 = (10^3\ m)^3 = 10^9\ m^3 = 1\ 000\ 000\ 000$ cubic metres (*not* $1\ k(m)^3 = 10^3\ m^3 = 1\ 000$ cubic metres). Similarly, $1\ cm^2$ (1 square centimetre) $= (10^{-2}\ m)^2 = 10^{-4}\ m^2 = 0,000\ 1\ m^2$, and $1\ \mu s^{-1}$ (1 reciprocal microsecond) $= (10^{-6}\ s)^{-1} = 10^6\ s^{-1} = 1\ 000\ 000$ per second.

It will be noticed that one SI base unit, the kilogram, has a prefix in its name. This is for historical reasons. The CIPM has decided that the names of decimal multiples and submultiples of the kilogram are formed by adding appropriate prefixes to the word "gram".

The units that are formed by means of prefixes should not be called SI units: the SI units are confined to the base, derived, and supplementary units, which form a coherent set. The result of using a prefix is a *multiple (or submultiple) of an SI unit.*

Compound prefixes must not be used. Example: use nano-metre, nm (not "millimicrometre", mμm).

Non-SI units

A few non-SI units are so widely used that they are part of our everyday lives, and in adopting the SI the CGPM retained eight such units for general use with the SI; they are listed in Table 5.

Table 5. Non-SI units retained for general use with the SI

Quantity	Unit	Symbol for unit	Value in SI units
time	minute	min	60 s
	hour	h	3 600 s
	day	d	86 400 s
plane angle	degree	°	$\pi/180$ rad
	minute	'	$\pi/10\,800$ rad
	second	''	$\pi/648\,000$ rad
volume	litre	l	$1\ dm^3 = 10^{-3}\ m^3$
mass	tonne	t	1 000 kg

Some of these units, particularly the litre and the units of time, are of great importance in the health professions. It should be explained that the litre is a "special name" given to the sub-multiple "cubic decimetre" of the SI unit of volume.[1] Similarly, "tonne"[2] is a special name given to a multiple of the SI unit of mass.

A further group of 12 non-SI units have been accepted by the CGPM for use with the SI for a limited time (the length of that time will depend on circumstances: some of the units are in very widespread use, some have already been largely superseded, and for some a time limit has been set by the relevant international organizations). The units of this group that may be of concern to the health professions are listed in Table 6.

The other five units of this group are the nautical mile (no symbol), 1 852 m; the knot (no symbol), approx. 0,514 m/s; the are (symbol: a), 100 m²; the hectare (symbol: ha), 10 000 m²; and the gal (symbol: Gal), 10^{-2} m/s².

Table 6. Non-SI units accepted for use for a limited time that are of concern in the health professions

Unit name	Unit symbol	Value in SI units
ångström	Å	10^{-10} m (0,1 nm)
barn	b	10^{-28} m² (100 fm²)
bar	bar	100 000 Pa (0,1 MPa)
normal atmosphere	atm	101 325 Pa
curie	Ci	$3,7 \times 10^{10}$ Bq (or $3,7 \times 10^{10}$ s^{-1})
röntgen	R	$2,58 \times 10^{-4}$ C/kg
rad	rad or rd[a]	10^{-2} Gy (or 10^{-2} J/kg)

[a] Symbol rd if there is any danger of confusion with the symbol rad for radian.

[1] It has often been asserted in the medical literature that the litre is "the fundamental SI unit of volume". This in untrue; the misunderstanding arises from the fact that the litre has been widely adopted by the health professions as the unit of volume to be used with the SI in those professions. (It should also be reiterated that there are no "fundamental" units in the SI: see footnote 3, page 7.)
[2] The commonly used term "metric ton" is a misnomer.

Finally, the CGPM has retained four non-SI units for use with the SI in specialized fields: the electronvolt (symbol: eV), the unified atomic mass unit (symbol: u), the parsec (symbol: pc), and the astronomic unit (symbol in the English language: AU). None of these is of concern in general medical practice (although the electronvolt is used in radiology and allied fields).

Writing of symbols and numbers [1]

Rules for the writing of symbols for units have been given in several places in the preceding text, where appropriate. A few additional rules are given here, together with the rules for writing numbers.

Symbols for units are always written in roman (upright) type, even if they occur in text that is set in italics. (On the other hand, symbols for quantities—see footnote 4 on page 7—are printed in italics, even if they occur in italic text; they are not part of the SI and are not dealt with in this book.)

Symbols for units do not change in the plural. Example: five kilometres is written 5 km, not 5 kms.

Symbols for units are never followed by a full stop (period), unless they occur at the end of a sentence. Examples: 5 g (not 5 g.); 10 ml (not 10 ml.).

In writing numbers, either a comma or a dot *on the line* may be used as the decimal marker in English text, but a dot on the line should not be used as the decimal marker in any text in which this symbol is used to indicate·multiplication. (In languages other than English, only the comma is used.) Most international bodies have indicated a preference for the use of the comma. A raised dot (for example, 5·2) should never be used (the raised dot is reserved as a symbol to indicate multiplication).

Digits should be separated (by small spaces) into groups of three to left and right of the decimal marker. No punctuation of any kind should separate the group of digits. Examples:

Correct: 1 000,350 1   ("one thousand point [or comma] three
1 000.350 1   five zero one")
0,562 013 ("zero point [or comma] five six two
0.562 013 zero one three")

Incorrect: 1,000.350,1
1'000,350'1
0.562,013
0,562'013

[1] Some of these rules were adopted by the Conférence générale des Poids et Mesures, and others were originally devised by the International Organization for Standardization; they are reproduced in the BIPM publications listed in Appendix 3.

2. Practical application

Although the number of "new" units involved in the change to the SI in general medical practice is small, several important factors are involved in their practical application. The recommendations of the competent international bodies on these matters are summarized in the following pages.

The mole

The use of the SI, which includes a unit of "amount of substance", implies the use of that unit (the **mole**) rather than mass units for all substances whose relative molecular mass [1] is known, and this has been made explicit by virtually all the relevant international organizations [2] and is implicit in resolution WHA30.39 to which reference has been made earlier. The consequences are described below.

Amount of substance

"Amount of substance" units (the mole or a submultiple thereof) will replace mass units such as the gram and milligram wherever possible.

Concentration

The term "concentration" has little meaning when used alone, since concentration can be expressed in many different ways. The unqualified term should therefore be avoided; instead, the correct quantity name, as given in Table 7, should be used. All these quantities are used in clinical chemistry, although some are used far more than others. The choice of units for concentration quantities involves the important principle that, in all the units listed in the last column of Table 7, the numerator may be changed to a multiple or submultiple, but the denominator should never be changed. Thus molality may be expressed in mmol/kg (instead of mol/kg), but not in µmol/g; substance fraction (mole fraction) may be expressed in mmol/mol (instead of mol/mol), but not in µmol/mmol. In all derived units whose denominator is a volume unit, only the litre should be used as the denominator

---

[1] Formerly called "molecular weight", but this term is incorrect since it means the weight (really the mass) of a molecule, and what is intended is the *relative* mass of a molecule with respect to the mass of an atom of hydrogen (strictly speaking this definition is not fully accurate, but it will serve for practical purposes). This quantity is, therefore, a ratio, and not a mass ("weight") at all.

[2] For example, the International Committee for Standardization in Hematology (of the International Society of Hematology), the International Federation of Clinical Chemistry, and the International Union of Pure and Applied Chemistry (Section on Clinical Chemistry).

(submultiple denominators such as the decilitre, dl, should not be used). Thus mass concentration may be expressed in g/l or mg/l (instead of kg/l), but not in g/dl or mg/dl. (The use of a single, unvarying denominator renders numerical values immediately comparable and prevents errors of interpretation that can occur all too easily when a variety of denominators—e.g., millilitre, decilitre, and litre—are used, as was the case in the past.)

Substance concentration. Concentration of substances whose relative molecular mass is known [1] are expressed in terms of *substance concentration* [2]—that is, in terms of mole (or a submultiple such as millimole or nanomole) per litre. As was mentioned above, the litre is the preferred denominator, and not some other volume such as the decilitre (100 ml).

Substance concentration should never be referred to as "molar concentration" or "molarity". In chemistry, the internationally agreed meaning of the adjective "molar" is *divided by amount of substance* [3]—i.e., *divided by mole*—and since substance concentration is mole divided by litre (mol/l), the term cannot be applied to it. The term "molarity" is deprecated and should not be used for any purpose. The symbol M should not be used instead of mol/l (nor should mM, nM, etc. be used for mmol/l, nmol/l, etc.).

When the mole is used, the entities involved must be specified. One can have, for example, a mole of molecules, of atoms, of ions, or of electrons. Since a laboratory report stating "glucose, substance concentration x mmol/l" clearly refers to molecules, these need not be specified. But a report stating "potassium, substance concentration x mmol/l" would be incomplete, since it is potassium *ion* that is measured (although it is unlikely that such a report would be misinterpreted); to be strictly correct, the report should read "potassium ion, substance concentration x mmol/l". (This example also illustrates the rule that the quantity name should always be given; the unit alone is not sufficient to avoid ambiguity. For example, "potassium ion, x mmol/l" could mean x millimoles per litre of solvent; but the inclusion of the quantity name "substance concentration" makes it clear that the report means x millimoles per litre of solution.)

---

[1] Under certain circumstances, it is possible to apply substance concentration to substances, for instance proteins, whose relative molecular mass is unknown or uncertain, as for example when the molecule of such a substance contains a metal atom (e.g., the iron atom in hemoglobin). By determining the amount of the metal that is present (e.g., the amount of iron in blood), which can be done with great accuracy, the substance concentration of the molecule can be measured, despite the fact that its relative molecular mass may not be accurately known. Similar considerations apply to a number of substances, including enzymes.

[2] An abbreviated form of the strictly correct "amount of substance concentration".

[3] Or, in a few cases, "divided by substance concentration".

Table 7. Concentration quantities and units[a]

Name of quantity	Definition	Unit[b]
substance concentration [of a given solute component]	amount of substance of a solute divided by volume of solution	(mol/m^3); mol/l
molality [of a given solute component]	amount of substance of a solute divided by mass of solvent	mol/kg
mole fraction (or substance fraction) [of a given component]	amount of substance of a component divided by amount of substance of mixture (i.e., all components of the system)	mol/mol
mole ratio (or substance ratio) [of a given solute component]	amount of substance of a solute divided by amount of substance of the solvent	mol/mol
mass concentration [of a given component]	mass of a component (e.g., solute) divided by volume of system (e.g., solution)	(kg/m^3); kg/l
mass fraction [of a given component]	mass of a component divided by mass of system (mixture)	kg/kg
volume fraction [of a given component]	volume of a component divided by volume of system (mixture)	(m^3/m^3); l/l
number concentration[c]	number of specified particles or elementary entities divided by volume of system (mixture)	(m^{-3}); l^{-1}
number fraction[d]	number of specified particles or elementary entities divided by total number of particles or entities in the system (mixture)	1 (a ratio)
substance content[e] [of a given component]	amount of substance of a component divided by mass of system (mixture)	mol/kg

[a] The table is limited to the quantities and units likely to be encountered in general medical practice. Additional quantities and units will be necessary in certain specialties, such as radiation medicine.

[b] Units not enclosed within parentheses are those that will normally be used in medical practice (but see the text with respect to the use of submultiple numerators). Where these units differ from the corresponding SI units, the latter are given within parentheses. It should be noted that if submultiple numerators are not used, some of the units listed (mol/mol, kg/kg, l/l) are simple ratios—i.e., the unit is "1".

[c] For example, the number of specified molecules in a mixture divided by the volume of the mixture ("molecular concentration").

[d] The quantity mole fraction (or substance fraction) is preferred whenever it is possible to use it.

[e] Not to be confused with molality.

Mass concentration. There are a few components of body fluids that cannot at present be measured in terms of amount of substance, owing to uncertainty regarding their relative molecular mass (and lack of another measurable molecular characteristic that could be used instead; see footnote 1, page 16). Such components will, for the time being, be reported in terms of mass concentration (or, in some cases, mass fraction). In mass concentration units the litre is again the denominator, and not some other volume such as the decilitre.

Immunoglobulins other than IgG (formerly termed "gamma-globulin") will have to be reported in terms of mass concentration for the time being (and so, consequently, will "total" protein). Although it is possible to report IgG and albumin in terms of substance concentration, and some laboratories will do (or are already doing) so, many laboratories will prefer to use mass concentration until it is possible to report *all* proteins in terms of substance concentration. On the other hand, the expression of albumin in terms of substance concentration can convey important information (e.g., its physiological relationship to bilirubin). Other components that many laboratories will report in terms of mass concentration for the time being include ceruloplasmin and haptoglobin (however, since the latter is usually measured as hemoglobin-binding capacity, it should be expressed in the same units as hemoglobin).

Hemoglobin. Although hemoglobin can readily be expressed in terms of substance concentration, the International Committee for Standardization in Hematology (of the International Society of Hematology) has recommended that it should preferably be reported in terms of mass concentration, in grams per litre (g/l), pending clarification of the position regarding plasma proteins. The Committee has, however, said that substance concentration (in millimoles per litre, mmol/l) may be used provided it is specified whether the monomer—Hb(Fe)—or the tetramer— Hb(4Fe) —is used.[1] In practice, therefore, values will be quoted in either of the following two forms: (*a*) Hemoglobin, mass concentration *x* g/l or (*b*) Hemoglobin(Fe), substance concentration *y* mmol/l (or Hemoglobin(4Fe), substance concentration *z* mmol/l). (If mass concentration is used, numerical values will be 10 times greater than those in the former unit g/100 ml.)

Hydrogen ion concentration. Some laboratories will report hydrogen ion concentration in terms of substance concentration (e.g., in nmol/l) instead of pH. Although the pH scale is not inconsistent with the SI, it is based on a logarithmic relationship,[2]

---

[1] The inclusion in this book of a table based on the monomer does not imply that WHO recommends the use of the monomer in preference to the tetramer.

[2] pH is defined as the negative logarithm of activity.

and the use of substance concentration, which avoids this complication, offers a number of advantages. However, the matter is still under study by the relevant international bodies, and no definitive recommendation has yet been made. Consequently, no recommendation is made in this book and a table of equivalent values in pH and in hydrogen ion concentration is not included.

Enzymes. The SI unit of catalytic activity (formerly termed enzymic activity) is mole per second (mol·s^{-1} or mol/s).[1] IUPAC has provisionally approved the special name katal (symbol: kat) for this unit (i.e., 1 kat = 1 mol/s), and this name has also been approved by the IUB-IUPAC Joint Commission on Biochemical Nomenclature. However, the katal has not yet been approved by CGPM and it is not, therefore, an SI unit. The mole per second (and the katal if approved) will replace the old international enzyme unit (symbol: U). The conversion factors are as follows: 1 U = 1 μmol/min = 16,67 nmol/s = 16,67 nkat (nkat = nano-katal). Since there is as yet no definitive recommendation on the subject, and the katal is not yet an SI unit, conversion factors for enzyme units are not included in Part 5 of this book.

Urine analyses

The result of analyses of urine may be expressed in terms of *substance flux*—i.e., amount of substance excreted divided by time (e.g., nmol/s). In practice, however, most of them are usually expressed in terms of total daily excretion, in amount of substance units (a multiple of the mole).

Pharmaceuticals

In the pharmaceutical field the changes involved in the use of SI units are relatively minor. In a few countries units such as the ounce, the grain, the dram, the minim, and the fluid ounce will be replaced by the SI units of mass and volume, but the great majority of countries already use the latter for the preparation of medicaments (e.g., the compounding of prescriptions). The main change will be the use of the mole.

Dosages of drugs and concentrations of solutions for administration to patients should always be indicated (a) unambiguously and (b) in such a way as will be most useful to those who administer or prescribe them.

Since, in using the SI, the concentration of most body-fluid constituents is expressed as substance concentration, this implies that the concentration of solutions for administration orally, intravenously, or by some other route should be expressed

---

[1] This refers to the amount of substrate transformed per second as a result of catalysis. The katal is therefore that amount of enzyme that catalyses the transformation of substrate at the rate of 1 mol/s.

in the same manner. For example, plasma (or serum) chloride and glucose levels are expressed in millimoles per litre (mmol/l), and sodium chloride and glucose solutions for intravenous administration should be labelled similarly. In many cases, however, the use of mass units in addition to amount of substance or substance concentration units will be advisable or even necessary.

The pascal

Blood gases

The partial pressures of blood gases (pO_2 and pCO_2) will normally be expressed in terms of the kilopascal (kPa) instead of the millimetre of mercury (mmHg).

Blood pressure, etc.

The change to the pascal for measuring other physiological pressures (e.g., blood pressure, cerebrospinal fluid pressure, intraocular pressure) will necessarily be gradual. The World Health Assembly resolution called for pressure-measuring instruments such as sphygmomanometers to carry scales in both kilopascals and millimetres of mercury (or centimetres of water, as appropriate) "for the time being... pending wider adoption of the use of the pascal in other [i.e., nonmedical] fields". During a thorough discussion of the subject, the delegates to the Health Assembly expressed the desire that both units be used side by side for a period in order to accustom members of the health professions to the new unit. It is suggested that the best way to do this would be (taking arterial blood pressure as an example) to quote values in kilopascals followed by the equivalent in millimetres of mercury within parentheses for a few years, thus: 16 kPa (120 mmHg). Finally, the use of the mmHg would be dropped completely.

The joule

The use of SI units involves the replacement of the so-called "calorie" by the **joule**. In fact, there is no such unit as the "calorie", and the correct name for the unit that has been used in nutrition and for the calculation of energy is the thermochemical calorie (symbol: cal_{th}, not cal).[1] In nutrition, the unit used in the past was

---

[1] There has been great confusion over the nutritionists' "calorie" and numerous different values for it, and definitions of it, will be found in the literature. Contrary to what most textbooks state, the thermochemical calorie has been defined solely in terms of the joule since 1935.

in fact usually the thermochemical kilocalorie, often referred to simply as the "calorie", the "Calorie", or the "large calorie". The use of the joule will eliminate this confusion.

The principal obstacle to the use of the joule alone in *nutrition* is the fact that dietary tables giving values in joules are not yet widely available. As an interim measure, therefore, it is preferable that values be quoted in both joules and thermochemical calories pending the availability of such tables. In practice, either of the multiples kilojoule or megajoule will be used. It is recommended that, in general, the megajoule be used rather than the kilojoule in nutrition, in order to avoid excessively large numerical values. Values would therefore be quoted as follows: 5,69 MJ (1 360 kcal$_{th}$).

In *physiology,* the joule is the unit of both energy and quantity of heat. The joule also replaces the kilopond metre (kp·m) and the kilogram-force metre (kgf·m) as the unit of work.

Other units in physiology

The SI unit the **newton** replaces the kilopond (kp) and the kilogram-force (kgf) as the unit of force, and the **watt** replaces the kilopond metre per minute (kp·m/min) and the kilogram-force metre per minute (kgf·m/min) as the unit of power. (In physiological studies, particularly those involving bicycle ergometer tests, the latter quantity has often been called "work". This is incorrect usage, since what is measured is not an amount of work but the amount of work done divided by time—i.e., the rate of doing work—for which the correct name is power.)

As the unit of vascular resistance, the **kilopascal second per litre** (kPa·s/l) replaces both the millimetre of mercury minute per litre (mmHg·min/l) and the dyne second per centimetre to the fifth power (dyn·s/cm^5). For the measurement of airway resistance, the kilopascal second per litre also replaces the centimetre of water second per litre (cmH$_2$O · s/l).

Numerous other units are used in different branches of physiology, but the majority of them pertain to research rather than clinical practice, and the physiologist should have no difficulty in working out, on the basis of the description of the SI in Part 1, the appropriate SI derived unit for a given application.

The kelvin and the degree Celsius

The **kelvin** will probably have few applications in general medical practice (although it is of importance in some fields of medical research). Instead, the health professions will use the unit of Celsius temperature, the **degree Celsius,** which has been accepted by the CGPM. The unit degree Celsius is equal to the unit kelvin (but a given temperature does not have the same numerical value on the two scales: temperature in K equals temperature in °C plus 273,15—e.g., 0 °C = 273,15 K). It should be noted that the unit is degree Celsius, not degree centigrade. The symbol for degree Celsius is °C, and the two parts of the symbol are inseparable; the sign ° by itself properly means angular degree. Thus it is incorrect to write a Celsius temperature range as 37°-38 °C; on the other hand "37-38 °C", "37 °C-38 °C", and "37 °C to 38 °C" are correct. In writing a Celsius temperature, there should be a small space between the numerical value and the ° sign, but none between the latter and the C. Thus 37 °C is correct, but 37° C is incorrect. In measuring the Celsius temperature of the human body, expression to the nearest 0,1 °C is sufficient.

Radiation units

In radiology and allied fields, the joule per kilogram replaces the rad and the rem; the reciprocal second replaces the curie; and the **coulomb per kilogram** replaces the röntgen. However, in 1975 the CGPM adopted, at the request of the International Commission on Radiation Units and Measurements (ICRU), the **gray** (symbol: Gy) as a special name for the joule per kilogram for the measurement of absorbed dose. It added a note to the effect that the gray could also be used for other physical quantities in the field of ionizing radiation that are expressed in joule per kilogram. This means that absorbed dose index, kerma, and specific energy imparted are also expressed in terms of the gray (as listed in Table 3). Also in 1975, the CGPM adopted the **becquerel** (symbol: Bq) as a special name for the reciprocal second for the measurement of activity. No special name was adopted for the coulomb per kilogram. Following these CGPM decisions, ICRU recommended that the units curie, rad, and röntgen be abandoned and replaced by the SI units over a period of not less than 10 years (i.e., the old units should not be completely abandoned before 1985). At the same time it requested all international and national organizations to assist in implementing the change.

The present situation is summarized in Table 8. It is recommended that, as an interim measure, numerical values should, for most purposes, be quoted in the literature as in the examples in the right-hand column of this table. Attention is drawn to the recommendation that, in order to avoid confusion, dose equivalent (for which the old unit was the rem) should be expressed in **joule per kilogram**, and not gray. [1]

[1] The Comité consultatif des Unités (see footnote 1, page 7) and ICRU have recommended that the use of the gray should be limited to the quantities mentioned in Tables 3 and 8, and the gray is so listed in the BIPM's official publication on the SI (ref. 1 and 2 in Appendix 3) (there has, however, not yet been time for the CGPM to act formally on this recommendation). It has been suggested that "sievert" (with the symbol Sv) be used as a special name for the joule per kilogram for the measu-

Table 8. Radiation quantities and units

Quantity	SI unit	Old unit	Example
absorbed dose; absorbed dose index; kerma; specific energy imparted	gray	rad	15 µGy (1,5 mrad)
absorbed dose rate	gray per second	rad per second	15 µGy/s (1,5 mrad/s)
dose equivalent	joule per kilogram	rem	10 mJ/kg (1 rem)
activity	becquerel	curie	37 MBq (1 mCi)
exposure	coulomb per kilogram	röntgen	0,258 µC/kg (1 mR)
exposure rate	coulomb per kilogram second (or ampere per kilogram)	röntgen per second	0,258 µC/(kg · s) (1 mR/s)

---

rement of dose equivalent. However, this matter is still under consideration by the responsible international bodies. The name "sievert", not having been accepted by the CGPM, is therefore not part of the SI. Consequently it is recommended that, for the time being, numerical values for dose equivalent be given as in Table 8.

3. Standardized reporting of laboratory results

The SI specifies only the units and symbols, and in some cases the names of quantities, that are to be used, and not how results should be reported. However, particularly for the health professions, clarity in the reporting of results is essential, since the life of a patient may well depend on their accuracy and lack of ambiguity. The appropriate international bodies, IFCC and IUPAC, have made a number of recommendations for standardizing the way in which clinical chemistry results are reported. These recommendations include a number of names of quantities in addition to those specified in the SI. These names (both those that are specified in the SI itself and the additional ones recommended by IFCC and IUPAC) are used in Parts 4 and 5 of this book. The recommendations also include standard names for components.

To prevent ambiguity in laboratory reports, the following information should always be given.

(a) The system (e.g., the patient, whole blood, plasma, serum, urine).

(b) The component that was determined (e.g., creatinine, glucose).

(c) The quantity that was measured (e.g., substance concentration).

(d) The numerical value.

(e) The unit.

Abbreviations for use in clinical laboratory reporting

IFCC and IUPAC have recommended a number of abbreviations for the names of systems and quantities [1] that may be used in order to avoid excessively lengthy laboratory reports. These are meant for use only in clinical laboratory reports; for instance, they should not be used in writing scientific papers, when they might, indeed, lead to ambiguity. Furthermore, IFCC and IUPAC recommend that, even in laboratory reports, whenever there might be danger of misunderstanding the names should be written in full. For reasons of space it has been necessary to use these abbreviations in Parts 4 and 5 of this book. The principal abbreviations are listed below.

---

[1] There are also *symbols,* as distinct from abbreviations, for most of these quantities. They are not dealt with in this book but may be found in *A guide to international recommendations on names and symbols for quantities and on units of measurement,* Geneva, World Health Organization, 1975.

Abbreviations and codes for the system

a	(as prefix) arterial	Lkc	leukocyte
B	blood	Lkcs	leukocytes
d	(as prefix) day, 24 h	P	plasma
Erc	erythrocyte[1]	Pt	patient
Ercs	erythrocytes[1]	S	serum
f	(as prefix) fasting	Sf	spinal fluid
F	faeces	U	urine

These abbreviations may be combined as appropriate. Examples: aB, arterial blood; fPt, fasting patient; (B)Ercs, blood erythrocytes; dU, 24-hour urine; (fPt)P, plasma from a fasting patient.

Abbreviations for names of quantities

ams.	amount of substance	numfr.	number fraction
diff.	difference	rel.	relative
equil.	equilibration	substc.	substance concentration
massc.	mass concentration[2]	substfr.	substance fraction (mole
massfr.	mass fraction[2]		fraction)
molal.	molality	vol.	volume
numc.	number concentration	volfr.	volume fraction

Form of clinical laboratory reports

The recommendations of IFCC and IUPAC are that laboratory reports be written in the following form:
(1) the name of the system or its abbreviation;
(2) a dash (in typewriting, two hyphens);
(3) the name of the component (never abbreviated), with an initial capital letter;
(4) a comma;
(5) the quantity name, with an initial lower-case letter,[3] or its abbreviation;
(6) an "equals" sign;
(7) the numerical value and the unit.[4]

---

[1] Erc and Ercs represent recent recommendations. The abbreviations Ery and Erys, which were formerly recommended, will be found in numerous documents.
[2] The formerly recommended abbreviations were masc. and masfr.
[3] It must be emphasized that the quantity name must always be included: the unit alone is not sufficient.
[4] Strictly speaking, one should say "numerical value times unit" (since measured quantity = numerical value × unit), but the "times sign" (×) is not used in reporting.

Examples (in full and abbreviated):

Plasma from fasting patient—Glucose, substance concentration = 4,9 mmol/l

(fPt)P—Glucose, substc. = 4,9 mmol/l

Blood—Hemoglobin(Fe), substance concentration = 8,0 mmol/l

B—Hemoglobin(Fe), substc. = 8,0 mmol/l

Serum—Sodium ion, substance concentration = 142 mmol/l

S—Sodium ion, substc. = 142 mmol/l

24-h Urine—Glucose, amount of substance = 13,8 mmol

dU—Glucose, ams. = 13,8 mmol

4. Tables of equivalent values

Tables of equivalent values in "old" units and "new" units will be found for the following on the pages indicated:

The abbreviations in the *headings* of the tables indicate the system to which the numerical values in the table apply (P, plasma; S, serum; Sf, spinal fluid; dU, 24-hour urine). A combined abbreviation such as P,S indicates that the numerical values apply to either plasma or serum.

The *conversion factors* on which the tables of equivalent values are based are tabulated in Part 5.

Nomograms for some of the most important of the tests tabulated above are printed on the inside and outside of the back cover, for convenient quick reference. A nomogram for body temperature conversion (°C and °F) is included.

Throughout the tables, the "new" (SI) units and values are printed in **bold** type.

---

bilirubins, P,S

μmol/l	mg/dl	μmol/l	mg/dl	μmol/l	mg/dl
1	0,058	21	1,23	240	14,0
2	0,117	22	1,29	260	15,2
3	0,175	23	1,34	280	16,4
4	0,234	24	1,40	300	17,5
5	0,292	25	1,46	320	18,7
6	0,351	26	1,52	340	19,9
7	0,409	27	1,58	360	21,0
8	0,468	28	1,64	380	22,2
9	0,526	29	1,70	400	23,4
10	0,585	30	1,76	420	24,6
11	0,643	40	2,34		
12	0,702	60	3,51		
13	0,760	80	4,68		
14	0,819	100	5,85		
15	0,877	120	7,02		
16	0,935	140	8,19		
17	0,994	160	9,35		
18	1,05	180	10,5		
19	1,11	200	11,7		
20	1,17	220	12,9		

mg/dl	μmol/l	mg/dl	μmol/l	mg/dl	μmol/l
0,1	1,71	1,6	27,4	13,0	222
0,2	3,42	1,7	29,1	14,0	239
0,3	5,13	1,8	30,8	15,0	256
0,4	6,84	1,9	32,5	16,0	274
0,5	8,55	2,0	34,2	17,0	291
0,6	10,3	3,0	51,3	18,0	308
0,7	12,0	4,0	68,4	19,0	325
0,8	13,7	5,0	85,5	20,0	342
0,9	15,4	6,0	103	21,0	359
1,0	17,1	7,0	120	22,0	376
1,1	18,8	8,0	137	23,0	393
1,2	20,5	9,0	154	24,0	410
1,3	22,2	10,0	171	25,0	428
1,4	23,9	11,0	188		
1,5	25,6	12,0	205		

calcium(II), P,S

mmol/l	mg/dl	mmol/l	mg/dl	mmol/l	mg/dl
0,1	0,401	1,6	6,41	3,1	12,4
0,2	0,802	1,7	6,81	3,2	12,8
0,3	1,20	1,8	7,21	3,3	13,2
0,4	1,60	1,9	7,62	3,4	13,6
0,5	2,00	2,0	8,02	3,5	14,0
0,6	2,40	2,1	8,42		
0,7	2,80	2,2	8,82		
0,8	3,21	2,3	9,22		
0,9	3,61	2,4	9,62		
1,0	4,01	2,5	10,0		
1,1	4,41	2,6	10,4		
1,2	4,81	2,7	10,8		
1,3	5,21	2,8	11,2		
1,4	5,61	2,9	11,6		
1,5	6,01	3,0	12,0		

mg/dl	mmol/l	mg/dl	mmol/l	mg/dl	mmol/l
0,5	0,125	5,5	1,37	10,5	2,62
1,0	0,250	6,0	1,50	11,0	2,74
1,5	0,374	6,5	1,62	11,5	2,87
2,0	0,499	7,0	1,75	12,0	2,99
2,5	0,624	7,5	1,87	12,5	3,12
3,0	0,748	8,0	2,00	13,0	3,24
3,5	0,873	8,5	2,12	13,5	3,37
4,0	0,998	9,0	2,24	14,0	3,49
4,5	1,12	9,5	2,37		
5,0	1,25	10,0	2,50		

calcium(II), dU

mmol	mg	mmol	mg	mmol	mg
0,5	20,0	5,5	220	10,5	421
1,0	40,1	6,0	240	11,0	441
1,5	60,1	6,5	260	11,5	461
2,0	80,2	7,0	280	12,0	481
2,5	100	7,5	301	12,5	501
3,0	120	8,0	321	13,0	521
3,5	140	8,5	341	13,5	541
4,0	160	9,0	361	14,0	561
4,5	180	9,5	381	14,5	581
5,0	200	10,0	401	15,0	601

mg	5	10	15
mmol	0,125	0,250	0,374

mg	mmol	mg	mmol	mg	mmol
20	0,499	220	5,49	420	10,5
40	0,998	240	5,99	440	11,0
60	1,50	260	6,49	460	11,5
80	2,00	280	6,99	480	12,0
100	2,50	300	7,48	500	12,5
120	2,99	320	7,98	520	13,0
140	3,49	340	8,48	540	13,5
160	3,99	360	8,98	560	14,0
180	4,49	380	9,48	580	14,5
200	4,99	400	9,98	600	15,0

cholesterols, P,S

mmol/l	mg/dl	mmol/l	mg/dl
1,0	38,7	11,0	425
1,5	58,0	11,5	445
2,0	77,3	12,0	464
2,5	96,7	12,5	483
3,0	116	13,0	503
3,5	135	13,5	522
4,0	155	14,0	541
4,5	174	14,5	561
5,0	193	15,0	580
5,5	213	15,5	599
6,0	232	16,0	619
6,5	251	16,5	638
7,0	271	17,0	657
7,5	290	17,5	677
8,0	309	18,0	696
8,5	329		
9,0	348		
9,5	367		
10,0	387		
10,5	406		

mg/dl	mmol/l	mg/dl	mmol/l
20	0,517	320	8,28
40	1,03	340	8,79
60	1,55	360	9,31
80	2,07	380	9,83
100	2,59	400	10,3
120	3,10	420	10,9
140	3,62	440	11,4
160	4,14	460	11,9
180	4,65	480	12,4
200	5,17	500	12,9
220	5,69	520	13,4
240	6,21	540	14,0
260	6,72	560	14,5
280	7,24	580	15,0
300	7,76	600	15,5

creatinine, P,S

μmol/l	mg/dl	μmol/l	mg/dl	μmol/l	mg/dl
20	0,226	420	4,75	820	9,28
40	0,452	440	4,98	840	9,50
60	0,679	460	5,20	860	9,73
80	0,905	480	5,43	880	9,95
100	1,13	500	5,66	900	10,2
120	1,36	520	5,88	920	10,4
140	1,58	540	6,11	940	10,6
160	1,81	560	6,33	960	10,8
180	2,04	580	6,56	980	11,1
200	2,26	600	6,79	1000	11,3
220	2,49	620	7,01		
240	2,71	640	7,24		
260	2,94	660	7,46		
280	3,17	680	7,69		
300	3,39	700	7,92		
320	3,62	720	8,14		
340	3,85	740	8,37		
360	4,07	760	8,60		
380	4,30	780	8,82		
400	4,52	800	9,05		

mg/dl	μmol/l	mg/dl	μmol/l	mg/dl	μmol/l
0,25	22,1	5,25	464	10,25	906
0,50	44,2	5,50	486	10,5	928
0,75	66,3	5,75	508	10,75	950
1,00	88,4	6,00	530	11,0	972
1,25	110	6,25	552	11,25	994
1,50	133	6,50	575	11,5	1020
1,75	155	6,75	597	11,75	1040
2,00	177	7,00	619	12,0	1060
2,25	199	7,25	641	12,25	1080
2,50	221	7,50	663	12,5	1100
2,75	243	7,75	685		
3,00	265	8,00	707		
3,25	287	8,25	729		
3,50	309	8,50	751		
3,75	332	8,75	774		
4,00	354	9,00	796		
4,25	376	9,25	818		
4,50	398	9,50	840		
4,75	420	9,75	862		
5,00	442	10,0	884		

creatinine, dU

mmol	mg	mmol	mg	mmol	mg
0,5	56,6	8,0	905	15,5	1750
1,0	113	8,5	962	16,0	1810
1,5	170	9,0	1020	16,5	1870
2,0	226	9,5	1070	17,0	1920
2,5	283	10,0	1130	17,5	1980
3,0	339	10,5	1190	18,0	2040
3,5	396	11,0	1240	18,5	2090
4,0	452	11,5	1300	19,0	2150
4,5	509	12,0	1360	19,5	2200
5,0	566	12,5	1410		
5,5	622	13,0	1470		
6,0	679	13,5	1530		
6,5	735	14,0	1580		
7,0	792	14,5	1640		
7,5	848	15,0	1700		

mg	mmol	mg	mmol	mg	mmol
50	0,442	800	7,07	1550	13,7
100	0,884	850	7,51	1600	14,1
150	1,33	900	7,96	1650	14,6
200	1,77	950	8,40	1700	15,0
250	2,21	1000	8,84	1750	15,5
300	2,65	1050	9,28	1800	15,9
350	3,09	1100	9,72	1850	16,4
400	3,54	1150	10,2	1900	16,8
450	3,98	1200	10,6	1950	17,2
500	4,42	1250	11,0	2000	17,7
550	4,86	1300	11,5	2050	18,1
600	5,30	1350	11,9	2100	18,6
650	5,75	1400	12,4	2150	19,0
700	6,19	1450	12,8	2200	19,4
750	6,63	1500	13,3	2250	19,9

glucose, P,S,Sf

mmol/l	mg/dl	mmol/l	mg/dl	mmol/l	mg/dl
0,5	9,01	10,5	189	18,0	324
1,0	18,0	11,0	198	18,5	333
1,5	27,0	11,5	207	19,0	342
2,0	36,0	12,0	216	19,5	351
2,5	45,0	12,5	225	20,0	360
3,0	54,0	13,0	234	20,5	369
3,5	63,0	13,5	243	21,0	378
4,0	72,1	14,0	252	21,5	387
4,5	81,1	14,5	261	22,0	396
5,0	90,1	15,0	270	22,5	405
5,5	99,1	15,5	279	23,0	414
6,0	108	16,0	288	23,5	423
6,5	117	16,5	297	24,0	432
7,0	126	17,0	306	24,5	441
7,5	135	17,5	315	25,0	450
8,0	144				
8,5	153				
9,0	162				
9,5	171				
10,0	180				

mg/dl	mmol/l	mg/dl	mmol/l	mg/dl	mmol/l
10	0,555	210	11,6	360	20,0
20	1,11	220	12,2	370	20,5
30	1,66	230	12,8	380	21,1
40	2,22	240	13,3	390	21,6
50	2,78	250	13,9	400	22,2
60	3,33	260	14,4	410	22,8
70	3,88	270	15,0	420	23,3
80	4,44	280	15,5	430	23,9
90	5,00	290	16,1	440	24,4
100	5,55	300	16,6	450	25,0
110	6,10	310	17,2	460	25,5
120	6,66	320	17,8	470	26,1
130	7,22	330	18,3	480	26,6
140	7,77	340	18,9	490	27,2
150	8,33	350	19,4	500	27,8
160	8,88				
170	9,44				
180	9,99				
190	10,5				
200	11,1				

hemoglobin(Fe)

mmol/l	g/l	g/dl		mmol/l	g/l	g/dl
3,20	51,6	5,16		8,20	132	13,2
3,40	54,8	5,48		8,40	135	13,5
3,60	58,0	5,80		8,60	138	13,8
3,80	61,2	6,12		8,80	142	14,2
4,00	64,4	6,44		9,00	145	14,5
4,20	67,7	6,77		9,20	148	14,8
4,40	70,9	7,09		9,40	151	15,1
4,60	74,1	7,41		9,60	155	15,5
4,80	77,3	7,33		9,80	158	15,8
5,00	80,6	8,06		10,0	161	16,1
5,20	83,8	8,38		10,2	164	16,4
5,40	87,0	8,70		10,4	168	16,8
5,60	90,2	9,02		10,6	171	17,1
5,80	93,5	9,35		10,8	174	17,4
6,00	96,7	9,67		11,0	177	17,7
6,20	99,9	9,99		11,2	180	18,0
6,40	103	10,3		11,4	184	18,4
6,60	106	10,6		11,6	187	18,7
6,80	110	11,0		11,8	190	19,0
7,00	113	11,3		12,0	193	19,3
7,20	116	11,6		12,2	197	19,7
7,40	119	11,9		12,4	200	20,0
7,60	122	12,2		12,6	203	20,3
7,80	126	12,6		12,8	206	20,6
8,00	129	12,9		13,0	209	20,9

iron(III) (transferrin-bound), P,S

µmol/l	µg/dl	µmol/l	µg/dl	µmol/l	µg/dl
2	11,2	32	179	52	290
4	22,3	34	190	54	302
6	33,5	36	201	56	313
8	44,7	38	212	58	324
10	55,8	40	223	60	335
12	67,0	42	234	62	346
14	78,2	44	246	64	357
16	89,4	46	257	66	368
18	100	48	268	68	380
20	112	50	279	70	391
22	123				
24	134				
26	145				
28	156				
30	168				

µg/dl	µmol/l	µg/dl	µmol/l	µg/dl	µmol/l
10	1,79	160	28,6	310	55,5
20	3,58	170	30,4	320	57,3
30	5,37	180	32,2	330	59,1
40	7,16	190	34,0	340	60,9
50	8,95	200	35,8	350	62,7
60	10,7	210	37,6	360	64,5
70	12,5	220	39,4	370	66,2
80	14,3	230	41,2	380	68,0
90	16,1	240	43,0	390	69,8
100	17,9	250	44,8	400	71,6
110	19,7	260	46,6		
120	21,5	270	48,3		
130	23,3	280	50,1		
140	25,1	290	51,9		
150	26,8	300	53,7		

phosphate (inorganic), P,S

mmol/l	mg/dl	mmol/l	mg/dl	mmol/l	mg/dl
0,1	0,310	1,6	4,96	2,6	8,05
0,2	0,619	1,7	5,26	2,7	8,36
0,3	0,929	1,8	5,58	2,8	8,67
0,4	1,24	1,9	5,88	2,9	8,98
0,5	1,55	2,0	6,19	3,0	9,29
0,6	1,86	2,1	6,50	3,1	9,60
0,7	2,17	2,2	6,81	3,2	9,91
0,8	2,48	2,3	7,12	3,3	10,2
0,9	2,79	2,4	7,43	3,4	10,5
1,0	3,10	2,5	7,74	3,5	10,8
1,1	3,41				
1,2	3,72				
1,3	4,03				
1,4	4,34				
1,5	4,65				

mg/dl	mmol/l	mg/dl	mmol/l	mg/dl	mmol/l
0,25	0,081	4,00	1,29	7,75	2,50
0,50	0,161	4,25	1,37	8,00	2,58
0,75	0,242	4,50	1,45	8,25	2,66
1,00	0,323	4,75	1,53	8,50	2,74
1,25	0,404	5,00	1,61	8,75	2,82
1,50	0,484	5,25	1,69	9,00	2,90
1,75	0,565	5,50	1,78	9,25	2,99
2,00	0,646	5,75	1,86	9,50	3,07
2,25	0,726	6,00	1,94	9,75	3,15
2,50	0,807	6,25	2,02	10,0	3,23
2,75	0,888	6,50	2,10		
3,00	0,968	6,75	2,18		
3,25	1,05	7,00	2,26		
3,50	1,13	7,25	2,34		
3,75	1,21	7,50	2,42		

mmHg→kPa

mmHg	kPa	mmHg	kPa	mmHg	kPa
1	0,133	36	4,80	71	9,46
2	0,267	37	4,93	72	9,60
3	0,400	38	5,07	73	9,73
4	0,533	39	5,20	74	9,86
5	0,667	40	5,33	75	10,0
6	0,800	41	5,47	76	10,1
7	0,933	42	5,60	77	10,3
8	1,07	43	5,73	78	10,4
9	1,20	44	5,87	79	10,5
10	1,33	45	6,00	80	10,7
11	1,47	46	6,13	81	10,8
12	1,60	47	6,27	82	10,9
13	1,73	48	6,40	83	11,1
14	1,87	49	6,53	84	11,2
15	2,00	50	6,67	85	11,3
16	2,13	51	6,80	86	11,5
17	2,27	52	6,93	87	11,6
18	2,40	53	7,07	88	11,7
19	2,53	54	7,20	89	11,9
20	2,67	55	7,33	90	12,0
21	2,80	56	7,47	91	12,1
22	2,93	57	7,60	92	12,3
23	3,07	58	7,73	93	12,4
24	3,20	59	7,86	94	12,5
25	3,33	60	8,00	95	12,7
26	3,47	61	8,13	96	12,8
27	3,60	62	8,26	97	12,9
28	3,73	63	8,40	98	13,1
29	3,87	64	8,53	99	13,2
30	4,00	65	8,66	100	13,3
31	4,13	66	8,80	102	13,6
32	4,27	67	8,93	104	13,9
33	4,40	68	9,06	106	14,1
34	4,53	69	9,20	108	14,4
35	4,67	70	9,33	110	14,7

mmHg→kPa *(continued)*

mmHg	kPa	mmHg	kPa	mmHg	kPa
112	14,9	182	24,3	252	33,6
114	15,2	184	24,5	254	33,9
116	15,5	186	24,8	256	34,1
118	15,7	188	25,1	258	34,4
120	16,0	190	25,3	260	34,7
122	16,3	192	25,6	262	34,9
124	16,5	194	25,9	264	35,2
126	16,8	196	26,1	266	35,5
128	17,1	198	26,4	268	35,7
130	17,3	200	26,7	270	36,0
132	17,6	202	26,9	272	36,3
134	17,9	204	27,2	274	36,5
136	18,1	206	27,5	276	36,8
138	18,4	208	27,7	278	37,1
140	18,7	210	28,0	280	37,3
142	18,9	212	28,3	282	37,6
144	19,2	214	28,5	284	37,9
146	19,5	216	28,8	286	38,1
148	19,7	218	29,1	288	38,4
150	20,0	220	29,3	290	38,7
152	20,3·	222	29,6	292	38,9
154	20,5	224	29,9	294	39,2
156	20,8	226	30,1	296	39,5
158	21,1	228	30,4	298	39,7
160	21,3	230	30,7	300	40,0
162	21,6	232	30,9		
164	21,9	234	31,2		
166	22,1	236	31,5		
168	22,4	238	31,7		
170	22,7	240	32,0		
172	22,9	242	32,3		
174	23,2	244	32,5		
176	23,5	246	32,8		
178	23,7	248	33,1		
180	24,0	250	33,3		

kPa→mmHg

kPa	0,1	0,2	0,3	0,4	0,5	0,6	0,7	0,8	0,9
mmHg	0,750	1,50	2,25	3,00	3,75	4,50	5,25	6,00	6,75

kPa	mmHg	kPa	mmHg
1	7,50	21	158
2	15,0	22	165
3	22,5	23	172
4	30,0	24	180
5	37,5	25	188
6	45,0	26	195
7	52,5	27	202
8	60,0	28	210
9	67,5	29	218
10	75,0	30	225
11	82,5	31	232
12	90,0	32	240
13	97,5	33	248
14	105	34	255
15	112	35	262
16	120	36	270
17	128	37	278
18	135	38	285
19	142	39	292
20	150	40	300

cmH₂O → kPa

cmH₂O	kPa		cmH₂O	kPa
1	0,098		21	2,06
2	0,196		22	2,16
3	0,294		23	2,26
4	0,392		24	2,35
5	0,490		25	2,45
6	0,588		26	2,55
7	0,686		27	2,65
8	0,784		28	2,74
9	0,883		29	2,84
10	0,981		30	2,94
11	1,08		31	3,04
12	1,18		32	3,14
13	1,27		33	3,24
14	1,37		34	3,33
15	1,47		35	3,43
16	1,57		36	3,53
17	1,67		37	3,63
18	1,76		38	3,73
19	1,86		39	3,82
20	1,96		40	3,92

thyroxin ("T₄"), P,S

nmol/l	μg/dl		nmol/l	μg/dl
10	0,777		160	12,4
20	1,55		170	13,2
30	2,33		180	14,0
40	3,11		190	14,8
50	3,88		200	15,5
60	4,66		210	16,3
70	5,44		220	17,1
80	6,21		230	17,9
90	6,99		240	18,6
100	7,77		250	19,4
110	8,54		260	20,2
120	9,32			
130	10,1			
140	10,9			
150	11,6			

μg/dl	nmol/l		μg/dl	nmol/l
1	12,9		11	142
2	25,7		12	154
3	38,6		13	167
4	51,5		14	180
5	64,4		15	193
6	77,2		16	206
7	90,1		17	219
8	103		18	232
9	116		19	244
10	129		20	257

triglyceride, P,S
(as glycerol trioleate)

mmol/l	mg/dl	mmol/l	mg/dl	mmol/l	mg/dl
1	88,5	16	1420	26	2300
2	177	17	1500	27	2390
3	266	18	1590	28	2480
4	354	19	1680	29	2570
5	443	20	1770	30	2660
6	531	21	1860	31	2740
7	620	22	1950	32	2830
8	708	23	2040	33	2920
9	797	24	2120	34	3010
10	885	25	2210	35	3100
11	974				
12	1060				
13	1150				
14	1240				
15	1330				

mg/dl	mmol/l	mg/dl	mmol/l	mg/dl	mmol/l
100	1,13	1100	12,4	2100	23,7
200	2,26	1200	13,6	2200	24,8
300	3,39	1300	14,7	2300	26,0
400	4,52	1400	15,8	2400	27,1
500	5,65	1500	16,9	2500	28,2
600	6,78	1600	18,1	2600	29,4
700	7,90	1700	19,2	2700	30,5
800	9,03	1800	20,3	2800	31,6
900	10,2	1900	21,4		
1000	11,3	2000	22,6		

urate, P,S

μmol/l	mg/dl	μmol/l	mg/dl	μmol/l	mg/dl
25	0,420	525	8,82	900	15,1
50	0,840	550	9,25	925	15,6
75	1,26	575	9,67	950	16,0
100	1,68	600	10,1	975	16,4
125	2,10	625	10,5	1000	16,8
150	2,52	650	10,9	1025	17,2
175	2,94	675	11,3	1050	17,6
200	3,36	700	11,8	1075	18,1
225	3,78	725	12,2	1100	18,5
250	4,20	750	12,6	1125	18,9
275	4,62	775	13,0	1150	19,3
300	5,04	800	13,4	1175	19,8
325	5,46	825	13,9	1200	20,2
350	5,88	850	14,3	1225	20,6
375	6,30	875	14,7	1250	21,0
400	6,72				
425	7,14				
450	7,56				
475	7,98				
500	8,40				

mg/dl	μmol/l	mg/dl	μmol/l	mg/dl	μmol/l
0,5	29,7	8,0	476	15,5	922
1,0	59,5	8,5	506	16,0	952
1,5	89,2	9,0	535	16,5	981
2,0	119	9,5	565	17,0	1010
2,5	149	10,0	595	17,5	1040
3,0	178	10,5	625	18,0	1070
3,5	208	11,0	654	18,5	1100
4,0	238	11,5	684	19,0	1130
4,5	268	12,0	714	19,5	1160
5,0	297	12,5	744	20,0	1190
5,5	327	13,0	773	20,5	1220
6,0	357	13,5	803	21,0	1250
6,5	387	14,0	833		
7,0	416	14,5	862		
7,5	446	15,0	892		

Urea Tables

The tables for urea on the following pages require some explanation, since at first sight they may seem somewhat complicated. This is because in the past this component has sometimes been reported in terms of urea and sometimes in terms of urea nitrogen. Since it is now recommended that numerical values be reported in terms of urea, the tables give equivalent numerical values as follows.

Plasma or serum

Page 46, top: numerical values for **urea in mmol/l** with equivalent numerical values for (*a*) urea in mg/dl and (*b*) urea nitrogen in mg/dl

Page 46, bottom: numerical values for urea nitrogen in mg/dl with equivalent numerical values for **urea in mmol/l**

Urine

Page 47, top: numerical values for **urea in mmol** with equivalent numerical values for (*a*) urea in g and (*b*) urea nitrogen in g

Page 47, middle: numerical values for urea in g with equivalent numerical values for **urea in mmol/l**

Page 47, bottom: numerical values for urea nitrogen in g with equivalent numerical values for **urea in mmol**

urea, P,S

urea mmol/l	urea, mg/dl	urea N, mg/dl		urea, mmol/l	urea, mg/dl	urea N, mg/dl
1	6,00	2,80		26	156	72,8
2	12,0	5,60		27	162	75,6
3	18,0	8,40		28	168	78,4
4	24,0	11,2		29	174	81,2
5	30,0	14,0		30	180	84,0
6	36,0	16,8		31	186	86,8
7	42,0	19,6		32	192	89,6
8	48,0	22,4		33	198	92,4
9	54,0	25,2		34	204	95,2
10	60,0	28,0		35	210	98,0
11	66,1	30,8		36	216	101
12	72,1	33,6		37	222	104
13	78,1	36,4		38	228	106
14	84,1	39,2		39	234	109
15	90,1	42,0		40	240	112
16	96,1	44,8		41	246	115
17	102	47,6		42	252	118
18	108	50,4		43	258	120
19	114	53,2		44	264	123
20	120	56,0		45	270	126
21	126	58,8		46	276	129
22	132	61,6		47	282	132
23	138	64,4		48	288	134
24	144	67,2		49	294	137
25	150	70,0		50	300	140

urea N, mg/dl	1	2	3	4
urea, mmol/l	0,357	0,714	1,07	1,43

urea N, mg/dl	urea mmol/l		urea N, mg/dl	urea, mmol/l		urea N, mg/dl	urea, mmol/l
5	1,78		55	19,6		100	35,7
10	3,57		60	21,4		105	37,5
15	5,36		65	23,2		110	39,3
20	7,14		70	25,0		115	41,0
25	8,92					120	42,8
			75	26,8			
30	10,7		80	28,6		125	44,6
35	12,5		85	30,3		130	46,4
40	14,3		90	32,1		135	48,2
45	16,1		95	33,9		140	50,0
50	17,8						

urea, dU

urea, mmol	urea, g	urea N, g	urea, mmol	urea, g	urea N, g
20	1,20	0,560	320	19,2	8,96
40	2,40	1,12	340	20,4	9,52
60	3,60	1,68	360	21,6	10,1
80	4,80	2,24	380	22,8	10,6
100	6,00	2,80	400	24,0	11,2
120	7,21	3,36	420	25,2	11,8
140	8,41	3,92	440	26,4	12,3
160	9,61	4,48	460	27,6	12,9
180	10,8	5,04	480	28,8	13,4
200	12,0	5,60	500	30,0	14,0
220	13,2	6,16	520	31,2	14,6
240	14,4	6,72	540	32,4	15,1
260	15,6	7,28	560	33,6	15,7
280	16,8	7,84	580	34,8	16,2
300	18,0	8,40	600	36,0	16,8

urea, g	urea, mmol	urea, g	urea, mmol	urea, g	urea, mmol
6	99,9	16	266	26	433
7	116	17	283	27	450
8	133	18	300	28	466
9	150	19	316	29	483
10	166	20	333	30	500
11	183	21	350	31	516
12	200	22	366	32	533
13	216	23	383	33	549
14	233	24	400	34	566
15	250	25	416	35	583

g urea N,	urea, mmol	urea N, g	urea, mmol	urea N, g	urea, mmol
0,5	17,8	5,5	196	10,5	375
1,0	35,7	6,0	214	11,0	393
1,5	53,6	6,5	232	11,5	410
2,0	71,4	7,0	250	12,0	428
2,5	89,2	7,5	268	12,5	446
3,0	107	8,0	286	13,0	464
3,5	125	8,5	303	13,5	482
4,0	143	9,0	321	14,0	500
4,5	161	9,5	339	14,5	518
5,0	178	10,0	357	15,0	536

5. Conversion Factors

The tables that follow give factors for converting numerical values in "old" units to numerical values in "new" (SI) units for (a) cell concentrations ("counts") and related quantities (page 51); (b) clinical chemistry determinations (pages 52-70); (c) quantities that are important in physiological tests (page 71); and (d) radiation quantities (page 71). A short list of miscellaneous units that should no longer be used is given on page 72.

Reference values are affected by many variables, including the procedure used in a given laboratory; the age, sex, and degree of physical activity of the subject; and climate. They should be established in consultation with a local laboratory. They have therefore not been included here, since it would have been misleading to do so in a book intended for worldwide use.

Notes on clinical chemistry table

The system involved (plasma, serum, urine, etc.) is listed in the first column. The second column gives the component that is determined and the name of the quantity that is measured (the abbreviations used for systems and quantities are explained on page 25). The component name is printed in **bold** type.[1] (In a few cases, names that are no longer recommended are also given in light-face type within square brackets, for identification.) The great majority of names in bold type are those that have been recommended internationally. In a few cases, however, a short-ened form of the recommended name has (for simplicity of presentation in the table) been used. In such cases the full name recommended by IFCC and IUPAC is given in a footnote. Certain changes in traditional names will be noticed. The most obvious is the listing of acids not as such but as "-ates". Thus ascorbic acid and ascorbate ion, salicylic acid and salicylate ion, and uric acid and urate ion are now reported as ascorbate, salicy-late, and urate, respectively. The conversion factors listed are based on the relative molecular masses of the undissociated acids.

A few of the component names in the second column are fol-lowed by numbers within parentheses, thus **fibrinogen(340 000).** These numbers, which are the relative molecular masses (M_r)

---

[1] In the past, practice with respect to the reporting of some components has varied in different areas, and occasionally it has been obscure. Plasma ammonia, for example, has been reported as N, as NH_3, or as NH_4^+. Such differences in practice tend to cause confusion. In the interests of the international comparability of information, it is desirable that the internationally recommended names of components listed in Part 5 be used.

of the components, form part of the component name (a) when the M_r is not exactly known (indicated by the sign $\sim$ before the numerical value in the last column), to indicate the M_r value used has the basis of the conversion factors (examples: albumin, ceruloplasmin, fibrinogen); and (b) when the component consists of a mixture, and the report is being made in terms of one of the constituents of the mixture (example: **tocopherol(417)** indicates that a number of different tocopherols may have been present in the sample, and that all are being reported as though they were 5,8-dimethyltocol, whose M_r is 417).

Elements are listed under their symbols rather than their names, the symbol being followed by the recommended name in bold type, thus:

Fe: **iron(III)**

(This arrangement is used solely in order to make it possible to use a single alphabetic order for the English and French editions of the table and thus avoid costly resetting of the type, greatly reducing the price of the book and the possibility of errors. It should not be used in laboratory reports.[1])

The word "method" within parentheses following a component name and an abbreviation for a quantity, thus:

haptoglobin, massc. (method)

indicates that it is essential to specify, in any laboratory report, the procedure that was used. (In the table, this is indicated only for those components for which it is *essential*. Many laboratories will feel it desirable to specify the method used for many additional components.)

For typographical reasons, component names are printed with initial lower-case letters. In laboratory reports, however (as previously noted), IFCC and IUPAC recommend the use of initial capital letters.

The third column lists the "old" or "traditional" unit. The fourth column ("Factor old →new") gives the factor by which numerical values in "old" units should be multiplied in order to convert them to numerical values in "new" units. The fifth column gives the "new" unit (in bold type).[2]

A figure 1 in the " 'New' unit" column indicates that the quantity involved is dimensionless and that values should be reported

---

[1] IFCC and IUPAC, however, recommend that symbols should be included *after* component names, to eliminate all possibility of ambiguity. Examples: **Calcium(II)(Ca); Phosphate(P, inorganic).**

[2] As noted in Part 1, multiples and submultiples should not be referred to as "SI units", and the litre is not an SI unit. The term " 'new' unit" is therefore used in column headings in order to avoid the use of a cumbersome expression such as "SI unit, multiple, or submultiple, or other unit approved for use with the SI".

The SI does not specify the particular submultiple of a unit that should be used for a given application, and submultiples other than those listed (in bold type) in the " 'New' unit" column may be used instead. Thus urine adrenaline, for which the "new unit" listed in the table is the nanomole, may also be reported in terms of the micromole. In general, however, use of the submultiples listed in the table will give numerical values of convenient size.

in decimal form (in such cases the unit, which is "unity" (1), is not given in a laboratory report). Example: phenolsulfonphthalein retention is reported as 0,25 (not 25%).

The conversion factor listed in italics to the right of the vertical line (in the "Factor new → old" column) is the factor by which numerical values in "new" units should be multiplied in order to convert them into numerical values in "old" units, if this should be necessary for any reason. [1]

The last column gives the relative atomic mass (A_r) or the relative molecular mass (M_r) of each element or compound.

*An asterisk in the clinical chemistry table indicates components for which detailed tables of equivalent values are given on pages 28-47.

**Two asterisks in the clinical chemistry table indicate components for which detailed tables of equivalent values are given on pages 28-47 and for which, in addition, nomograms are printed on the back cover.

Examples of how to use the tables

(a) *Converting numerical values in "old" units to numerical values in "new" units:*
        acetone 20,1 mg x 17,22 → acetone 346 µmol

(b) *Converting numerical values in "new" units to numerical values in "old" units:*
        acetone 346 µmol x 0,058 07 → acetone 20,1 mg

***

> Throughout the tables, the units printed in **bold** type are the "new" (SI) units.

---

[1] Large errors may arise if rounded-off numerical values in "x" units are converted, by the use of a rounded-off factor, into values in "y" units, which are then in turn rounded-off. Rounding-off should always be done at the last stage. For this reason, the tables give conversion factors to four significant figures.

Cell Concentrations
["Counts"] & Related Quantities

System	Component & quantity	"Old" unit	Factor old→new	"New" unit	Factor new→old
B	**coagulation,** time	min	1	**min**	1
		min	0,06	**ks**	16,67
B	**eosinophils,** numc.	µl⁻¹	0,001	**10⁹/l**	1 000
		10⁶/l	0,001	**10⁹/l**	1 000
(B)Erc (mean)	**erythrocyte,** vol. ["MCV"]	µ³	1	**fl**	1
B	**erythrocytes,** numc.	10⁶/µl	1	**10¹²/l**	1
		10⁶/mm³	1	**10¹²/l**	1
Sf	**erythrocytes,** numc.	µl⁻¹	1	**10⁶/l**	1
		mm⁻³	1	**10⁶/l**	1
B	**erythrocytes,** volfr. ["PCV"; "hematocrit"]	%	0,01	**1**	100
		ml/l	0,01	**1**	100
B	**leukocytes,** numc.	µl⁻¹	0,001	**10⁹/l**	1 000
		mm⁻³	0,001	**10⁹/l**	1 000
		10⁶/l	0,001	**10⁹/l**	1 000
Sf	**leukocytes,** numc.	µl⁻¹	1	**10⁶/l**	1
		mm⁻³	1	**10⁶/l**	1
(B)Lkcs	**leukocyte type,** numfr. ["differential count"]	%	0,01	**1**	100
(B)Ercs	**reticulocytes,**[a] numfr.	⁰/₀₀	1	**10⁻³**	1
		%	10	**10⁻³**	0,1
B	**reticulocytes,**[a] numc.			**10⁹/l**	
B	**thrombocytes,** numc.	µl⁻¹	0,001	**10⁹/l**	1 000
		mm⁻³	0,001	**10⁹/l**	1 000
		10⁶/l	0,001	**10⁹/l**	1 000

[a] Reticulocytes may be reported in terms of either number fraction ("per thousand") or number concentration (number x 10⁹/l).

See page 48 for explanation

Clinical Chemistry

System	Component & quantity	"Old" unit	Factor old→new	"New" unit	Factor new→old	M_r or A_r
dU	**acetone,** ams.	mg	17,22	**µmol**	0,058 08	58,079 8
	ACTH *see corticotropin*					
dU	**adrenaline,**[a] ams. (epinephrine)	µg	5,458	**nmol**	0,183 2	183,207
P,S	**albumin(69 000),** massc.	g/dl	10	**g/l**	0,1	~ 69 000
		g/l	1	**g/l**	1	
	substc.	g/dl	144,9	**µmol/l**	0,006 900	
		g/l	14,49	**µmol/l**	0,069 00	
dU	**aldosterone,** ams.	µg	2,774	**nmol**	0,360 4	360,449
P,S	**δ-aminolevulinate,** substc.	µg/dl	0,076 26	**µmol/l**	13,11	131,129
dU	**δ-aminolevulinate,** ams.	mg	7,626	**µmol**	0,131 1	131,129
P,S	**ammonium,**[b] substc.	µg/dl	0,587 2	**µmol/l**	1,703	$NH_3 = 17,030\,4$
		mg/l	58,72	**µmol/l**	0,017 03	
dU	**ammonium,**[b] ams.	mg	0,058 72	**mmol**	17,03	$NH_3 = 17,030\,4$

[a] The recommended name is **adrenalinium.**
[b] Includes ammonia + ammonium ion.

System	Component & quantity	"Old" unit	Factor old→new	"New" unit	Factor new→old	M_r or A_r
P	**androsterone**, substc.	µg/dl	34,43	**nmol/l**	0,029 04	290,445
P,S	**ascorbate**, substc. ("vitamin C")	mg/dl mg/l	56,78 5,678	**µmol/l** **µmol/l**	0,017 61 0,176 1	176,126
	BUN see urea					
	barbiturates[c]					
P,U	**allobarbital**, substc.	mg/dl mg/l	48,03 4,803	**µmol/l** **µmol/l**	0,020 82 0,208 2	208,216 4
P,U	**amobarbital**, substc.	mg/dl mg/l	44,19 4,419	**µmol/l** **µmol/l**	0,022 63 0,226 3	226,274 8
P,U	**aprobarbital**, substc.	mg/dl mg/l	47,57 4,757	**µmol/l** **µmol/l**	0,021 02 0,210 2	210,232 2
P,U	**barbital**, substc.	mg/dl mg/l	54,29 5,429	**µmol/l** **µmol/l**	0,018 42 0,184 2	184,194 4
P,U	**butalbital**, substc.	mg/dl mg/l	44,59 4,459	**µmol/l** **µmol/l**	0,022 43 0,224 3	224,259

[c]Some laboratories will not report individual barbiturates by name: in such cases, the component name is **barbiturate** (thus, P—Barbiturate, substc. = x µmol/l).

See page 48 for explanation

System	Component & quantity	"Old" unit	Factor old→new	"New" unit	Factor new→old	M_r or A_r
P,U	**pentobarbital**, substc.	mg/dl mg/l	44,19 4,419	µ**mol/l** µ**mol/l**	0,022 63 0,226 3	226,274 8
P,U	**phenobarbital**, substc.	mg/dl mg/l	43,06 4,306	µ**mol/l** µ**mol/l**	0,023 22 0,232 2	232,238 4
P,U	**secobarbital**, substc.	mg/dl mg/l	41,97 4,197	µ**mol/l** µ**mol/l**	0,023 83 0,238 3	238,285 8
aB	**base(H⁺ binding sites)**, substc. diff. ["base excess"]	meq/l	1	m**mol/l**	1	
	bicarbonate see carbonate + carbon dioxide; hydrogencarbonate					
P,S	****bilirubins**[d] [total], substc.	mg/dl mg/l	17,10 1,710	µ**mol/l** µ**mol/l**	0,058 47 0,584 7	584,671
S	Br: **bromide**, substc.	mg/dl	0,125 2	m**mol/l**	7,990	79,904
	bromsulphalein test see sulfobromophthaleinate					

[d] The plural form indicates bilirubin + derivatives (esters, conjugates).

See page 48 for explanation

System	Component & quantity	"Old" unit	Factor old→new	"New" unit	Factor new→old	M_r or A_r
P,S	*Ca: **calcium(II)**, substc.	meq/l mg/dl mg/l	0,5 0,249 5 0,024 95	**mmol/l** **mmol/l** **mmol/l**	2 4,008 40,08	40,08
dU	*Ca: **calcium(II)**, substc.	meq mg	0,5 0,024 95	**mmol** **mmol**	2 40,08	40,08
P,S	**carbonate**[e] + **carbon dioxide**, substc. ["bicarbonate"; "total CO_2"]	meq/l vol.%[f]	1 0,449 2	**mmol/l** **mmol/l**	1 2,226	
Gas(aB equil.)	**carbon dioxide**, partial pressure (37 °C) [pCO_2]	mmHg	0,133 3	**kPa**	7,502	
(B) Hb	**carboxyhemoglobin**, substfr.	%	0,01	**mol/mol** (= 1)	100	64 500
P	**carotenoids(537)**, substc.	µg/dl mg/dl mg/l	0,018 63 18,63 1,863	**µmol/l** **µmol/l** **µmol/l**	53,69 0,053 69 0,536 9	β-carotene = 536,882

catecholamines see
adrenaline ; noradrenaline

[e] "Carbonate" as a component includes carbonate, hydrogencarbonate, and carbonic acid, but not carbon dioxide.
[f] Carbon dioxide at 0 °C and 101,325 kPa ("STP").

System	Component & quantity	"Old" unit	Factor old→new	"New" unit	Factor new→old	M_r or A_r
S	**ceruloplasmin(160 000)**, massc. substc.	mg/dl mg/dl	10 0,062 50	**mg/l** **µmol/l**	0,1 16,00	~160 000
P,S	****cholesterols,** [g] substc.	mg/dl g/l	0,025 86 2,586	**mmol/l** **mmol/l**	38,67 0,386 7	386,660
P,S	Cl: **chloride**, substc.	meq/l mg/dl g/l	1 0,282 1 28,21	**mmol/l** **mmol/l** **mmol/l**	1 3,545 0,035 45	35,453
dU	Cl: **chloride**, ams.	meq g	1 0,282 1	**mmol** **mmol**	1 0,035 45	35,453
(B)Erc	**coproporphyrins(I + III),** substc.	µg/dl	15,27	**nmol/l**	0,065 47	654,718
dU	**coproporphyrins(I + III),** ams.	µg	1,527	**nmol**	0,654 7	654,718
P,S	**corticosteroid,** substc.	µg/dl	0,027 59	**µmol/l**	36,25	hydrocortisone = 362,465
P	**corticotropin,** substc. ["ACTH"]	pg/ml ng/l	0,220 2 0,220 2	**pmol/l** **pmol/l**	4,541 4,541	4 541,14

[g] The plural form indicates cholesterol + cholesterol esters.

System	Component & quantity	"Old" unit	Factor old→new	"New" unit	Factor new→old	M_r or A_r
	cortisol *see* corticosteroid					
S	**cortisone**, substc.	µg/dl	0,027 74	**µmol/l**	36,04	360,449
P	**creatine**, substc.	mg/dl	76,26	**µmol/l**	0,013 11	131,134
		mg/l	7,626	**µmol/l**	0,131 1	131,134
dU	**creatine**, ams.	mg	7,626	**µmol**	0,131 1	131,134
P,S	****creatinine**,[h] substc.	mg/dl	88,40	**µmol/l**	0,011 31	113,119
		mg/l	8,840	**µmol/l**	0,113 1	113,119
dU	***creatinine**,[h] ams.	mg	0,008 840	**mmol**	113,1	113,119
P,S	Cu: **copper(II)**, substc.	µg/dl	0,157 4	**µmol/l**	6,355	63,546
		mg/l	15,74	**µmol/l**	0,063 55	63,546
P,S	**cyanocobalamin**, substc. ["vitamin B-12"]	ng/dl	7,378	**pmol/l**	0,135 5	1 355,40
		ng/l	0,737 8	**pmol/l**	1,355	
		pg/ml	0,737 8	**pmol/l**	1,355	
S	**11-deoxycorticosteroid**, substc.	µg/dl	0,030 26	**µmol/l**	33,04	deoxycortico-sterone = 330,446

See page 48 for explanation

[h] Includes creatinine + creatininium ion. The recommended component name is **creatininium.**

System	Component & quantity	"Old" unit	Factor old→new	"New" unit	Factor new→old	M_r or A_r
	epinephrine see adrenaline					
dU	**estradiol**, ams.	µg	3,671	**nmol**	0,272 4	272,386
dU	**estriol**, ams.	µg	3,468	**nmol**	0,288 4	288,386
dU	**estrone**, ams.	µg	3,699	**nmol**	0,270 4	270,371
P,S	****Fe:iron(III)(Fe, transferrin-bound)**, substc.	µg/dl mg/l	0,179 1 17,91	**µmol/l** **µmol/l**	5,585 0,055 85	55,847
P	**fibrinogen(340 000)**, massc.	mg/dl g/dl	0,01 10	**g/l** **g/l**	100 0,1	~340 000
	substc.	mg/dl g/dl	0,029 41 29,41	**µmol/l** **µmol/l**	34,00 0,034 00	
P,S	**folates,**[i] substc.	µg/dl µg/l	22,66 2,266	**nmol/l** **nmol/l**	0,044 14 0,441 4	pteroylglutamic acid = 441,402
P,S	**galactose**, substc.	mg/dl mg/l	0,055 51 0,005 551	**mmol/l** **mmol/l**	18,02 180,2	180,157

The plural form indicates pteroylglutamic acid + derivatives (esters, conjugates).

System	Component & quantity	"Old" unit	Factor old→new	"New" unit	Factor new→old	M_r or A_r
	globulin *see* immunoglobulin					
P,S,Sf	**glucose**, substc.	mg/dl	0,055 51	**mmol/l**	18,02	180,157
		g/l	5,551	**mmol/l**	0,180 2	
dU	**glucose**, ams.	g	5,551	**mmol**	0,180 2	
S	**haptoglobin**, massc. (method)	mg/dl	0,01	**g/l**	100	∼ 100 000
S	**haptoglobin(Hb(4Fe)-binding sites)**, substc. (method)	mg/dl	0,155 1	**µmol/l**	6,446	Hb(4Fe) = 64 458
	hemiglobin *see* methemoglobin					
(B)Erc (mean)	**hemoglobin(Fe)**, ams. ["MCH"]	pg	0,062 06	**fmol**	16,11	Hb(4Fe) = 64 458
		µµg	0,062 06	**fmol**	16,11	
		γγ	0,062 06	**fmol**	16,11	
(B)Erc (mean)	**hemoglobin(Fe)**, substc. ["MCHC"]	g/dl	0,620 6	**mmol/l**	1,611	Hb(Fe) = 16 114,5
		g/l	0,062 06	**mmol/l**	16,11	
B	**hemoglobin(Fe)**, substc.	g/dl	0,620 6	**mmol/l**	1,611	Hb(Fe) = 16 114,5
		g/l	0,062 06	**mmol/l**	16,11	
		%	0,091 84	**mmol/l**	10,89	
	massc.	g/dl	10	**g/l**	0,1	(100% = 148 g/l)
		g/l	1	**g/l**	1	

See page 48 for explanation

— 59 —

System	Component & quantity	"Old" unit	Factor old→new	"New" unit	Factor new→old	M_r or A_r
B	Hg: **mercury(II)**, substc.	µg/l	4,985	**nmol/l**	0,200 6	200,59
dU	Hg: **mercury(II)**, ams.	µg	4,985	**nmol**	0,200 6	200,59
	5-HIA see 5-hydroxyindoleacetate					
dU	**hippurate**, ams.	g	5,581	**mmol**	0,179 2	N-benzoyl-glycine = 179,175
		mg	0,005 581	**mmol**	179,2	
	hydrocortisone see corticosteroid					
P	**hydrogencarbonate**, substc. ["standard bicarbonate"]	meq/l	1	**mmol/l**	1	
P	**3-hydroxybutyrate**, substc.	mg/dl	96,06	**µmol/l**	0,010 41	104,105
		mg/l	9,606	**µmol/l**	0,104 1	
dU	**17-hydroxycorticosteroid**, ams.	mg	2,759	**µmol**	0,362 5	hydrocortisone = 362,465
dU	**5-hydroxyindoleacetate**, ams.	mg	5,230	**µmol**	0,191 2	191,186
dU	**4-hydroxy-3-methoxymandelate**, ams. ["VMA"]	mg	5,046	**µmol**	0,198 2	198 157
dU	**hydroxyproline**, ams.	mg	7,626	**µmol**	0,131 1	131,131

System	Component & quantity	"Old" unit	Factor old→new	"New" unit	Factor new→old	M_r or A_r
P,S	l: **iodine(l, protein-bound)** ["PBI"]	µg/dl µg/l	78,80 7,880	**nmol/l** **nmol/l**	0,012 69 0,126 9	126,904
S	**immunoglobulin,**[j] massc.	mg/ml mg/dl g/dl	1 0,01 10	**g/l** **g/l** **g/l**	1 100 0,1	
P,S	**insulin,**[k] substc.	µg/l mU/l µU/ml	172,2 7,175 7,175	**pmol/l** **pmol/l** **pmol/l**	0,005 808 0,139 4 0,139 4	5 807,65

[j] With the exception of IgG (formerly termed "gamma-globulin"), immunoglobulins must for the time being be reported in terms of mass concentration. Most laboratories will therefore report all immunoglobulins in this manner. When numerical values are reported for individual immunoglobulins, the internationally recommended symbols IgA, IgG, IgM should be used.

[k] Insulin substance concentration is sometimes reported on the basis of $M_r = 5\,800$. In this case, the component name is **insulin(5 800)** and the conversion factors for "international units" (U) are based on the relationship 1 U = 41,67 µg) (conversion factors for individual are as follows:

Old unit	Factor old→new	New unit	Factor new→old
µg/l	172,4	pmol/l	0,005 800
mU/l	7,184	pmol/l	0,139 2
µU/ml	7,184	pmol/l	0,139 2

See page 48 for explanation

System	Component & quantity	"Old" unit	Factor old→new	"New" unit	Factor new→old	M_r or A_r
P,S	K: **potassium ion**, substc.	meq/l mg/l	1 0,025 58	**mmol/l** **mmol/l**	1 39,10	39,098
dU	K: **potassium ion**, ams.	meq g	1 25,58	**mmol** **mmol**	1 0,039 10	39,098
dU	**17-ketosteroids & ketogenic steroids**, ams.	mg	3,467	µmol	0,288 4	dehydro-epiandrosterone = 288,429
P	**lactate**, substc.	mg/dl mg/l	0,111 0 0,011 1	**mmol/l** **mmol/l**	9,008 90,08	90,079
P,S	Li: **lithium ion**, substc.	meq/l mg/dl mg/l	1 1,441 0,144 1	**mmol/l** **mmol/l** **mmol/l**	1 0,694 1 6,941	6,941
dF	**lipid** (total), mass	g	1	**g**	1	
P	**lipid** (total), massc.	mg/dl	0,01	**g/l**	100	
S	**lipoprotein**, massc. (method)	mg/dl	0,01	**g/l**	100	

System	Component & quantity	"Old" unit	Factor old→new	"New" unit	Factor new→old	M_r or A_r
B	**methemoglobin(Fe)**,[1] substc.	g/dl	620,6	**µmol/l**	0,001 611	16 114,5
	massc.	g/l	62,06	**µmol/l**	0,016 11	
		g/dl	10	**g/l**	0,1	
P,S	Mg: **magnesium(II)**, substc.	meq/l	0,5	**mmol/l**	2	24,305
		mg/dl	0,411 4	**mmol/l**	2,431	
		mg/l	0,041 14	**mmol/l**	24,31	
dU	Mg: **magnesium(II)**, ams.	meq	0,5	**mmol**	2	24,305
		mg	0,041 14	**mmol**	24,31	
P	**myoglobin**, substc.	mg/dl	0,584 8	**µmol/l**	1,710	17 100
		mg/l	0,058 48	**µmol/l**	17,10	
dU	**myoglobin**, ams.	mg	0,058 48	**µmol**	17,10	17 100
P	N: **amino-acid nitrogen**, substc.	mg/dl	0,713 9	**mmol/l**	1,401	14,006 7
		mg/l	0,071 39	**mmol/l**	14,01	
dU	N: **amino-acid nitrogen**, ams.	mg	0,071 39	**mmol**	14,01	14,006 7
	N, urea- see urea					

[1] The recommended component name is **hemiglobin(Fe)**.

See page 48 for explanation

System	Component & quantity	"Old" unit	Factor old→new	"New" unit	Factor new→old	M_r or A_r
P,S	Na: **sodium ion**, substc.	meq/l mg/dl g/l	1 0,435 0 43,50	**mmol/l** **mmol/l** **mmol/l**	1 2,299 0,022 99	22,989 8
dU	Na: **sodium ion**, ams.	meq g	1 43,50	**mmol** **mmol**	1 0,022 99	22,989 8
P,S	Ni: **nickel(II)**, substc.	µg/l	0,017 03	**µmol/l**	58,71	58,71
dU	**noradrenaline**,[m] substc. (norepinephrine)	µg	5,911	**nmol**	0,169 2	169,18
Gas(aB equil.)	**O₂: Oxygen**,[n] partial pressure (37 °C) ["pO_2"]	mmHg	0,133 3	**kPa**	7,502	
	O₂: oxygen saturation *see* oxyhemoglobin					
dU	**oxalate**, ams.	mg	7,932	**µmol**	0,126 1	oxalic acid dihydrate = 126,066
(B)Hb	**oxyhemoglobin**, substfr. ["oxygen saturation"]	%	0,01	**mol/mol** (= **1**)	100	

[m] The recommended name is **noradrenalinium**.
[n] The recommended name is **dioxygen**.

— 64 —

System	Component & quantity	"Old" unit	Factor old→new	"New" unit	Factor new→old	M_r or A_r
	PBI see I: iodine					
B	Pb: **lead(II)**, substc.	µg/dl	0,048 26	µ**mol/l**	20,72	207,2
		µg/l	0,004 826	µ**mol/l**	207,2	207,2
		mg/l	4,826	µ**mol/l**	0,207 2	
dU	Pb: **lead(II)**, ams.	µg	0,004 826	µ**mol**	207,2	207,2
		mg	4,826	µ**mol**	0,207 2	
Pt	**phenolsulfonphthaleinate**, rel. ams. (method) ["PSP test"]	%	0,01	**1**	100	
P,S	****phosphate(P, inorganic)**, substc.	mg/dl	0,322 9	**mmol/l**	3,097	P = 30,973 8
		mg/l	0,032 29	**mmol/l**	30,97	
dU	**phosphate(P, inorganic)**, ams.	mg	0,032 29	**mmol**	30,97	P = 30,973 8
P,S	**phospholipid**,° substc.	g/l	1,292	**mmol/l**	0,774 0	774
	— phosphorus	mg/dl	0,322 9	**mmol/l**	3,097	P = 30,973 8
		mg/l	0,032 29	**mmol/l**	30,97	P = 30,973 8
dU	**porphobilinogen**, ams.	mg	4,420	µ**mol**	0,226 2	226,232

° Numerical values may be reported as either phospholipid or phosphorus. The M_r listed (774) is the "mean".

See page 48 for explanation

System	Component & quantity	"Old" unit	Factor old→new	"New" unit	Factor new→old	M_r or A_r
dU	**pregnanediol**, ams.	mg	3,120	**μmol**	0,320 5	320,514
dU	**pregnanetriol**, ams.	mg	2,972	**μmol**	0,336 5	336,513
S	**progesterone**, substc.	μg/dl	31,80	**nmol/l**	0,031 45	314,467
		μg/l	3,180	**nmol/l**	0,314 5	
P,S,Sf,U	**protein**, massc.	g/dl	10	**g/l**	0,1	
		mg/dl	0,01	**g/l**	100	
(B)Erc	**protoporphyrin**, substc.	μg/dl	0,017 77	**μmol/l**	56,27	562,67
		μg/l	0,001 777	**μmol/l**	562,7	
	PSP see phenolsulfonphthaleinate					
P,B	**pyruvate**, substc.	mg/dl	113,6	**μmol/l**	0,008 806	88,063
		mg/l	11,36	**μmol/l**	0,088 06	
P,S	**retinol**, substc.	μg/dl	0,034 91	**μmol/l**	28,65	286,456
		μg/l	0,003 491	**μmol/l**	286,5	
P,S	**salicylate**, substc.	mg/dl	0,072 40	**mmol/l**	13,81	138,123
		mg/l	0,007 240	**mmol/l**	138,1	
	serotonin see 5-hydroxyindoleacetate					
	siderophilin see transferrin					

System	Component & quantity	"Old" unit	Factor old→new	"New" unit	Factor new→old	M_r or A_r
B	**sulfhemoglobin(Fe)**, substc.	g/dl	620,6	µmol/l	0,001 611	Hb(Fe) =
	massc.	g/l	62,06	µmol/l	0,016 11	16 114,5
		g/dl	10	g/l	0,1	
Pt	**sulfobromophthaleinate**, rel.	%	0,01	1	100	
	ams. (method) ["BSP test"]					
	sulfonamides[P]					
P,S	**sulfacetamide**, substc.	mg/dl	0,046 68	mmol/l	21,42	214,24
P,S	**sulfadiazine**, substc.	mg/dl	0,039 96	mmol/l	25,03	250,27
P,S	**sulfadimethoxine**, substc.	mg/dl	0,032 22	mmol/l	31,03	310,33
P,S	**sulfaguanidine**, substc.	mg/dl	0,046 68	mmol/l	21,42	214,24
P,S	**sulfamerazine**, substc.	mg/dl	0,037 84	mmol/l	26,43	264,30
P,S	**sulfamethizole**, substc.	mg/dl	0,036 99	mmol/l	27,03	270,32
P,S	**sulfamethoxazole**, substc.	mg/dl	0,039 48	mmol/l	25,33	253,28
P,S	**sulfanilamide**, substc.	mg/dl	0,058 07	mmol/l	17,22	172,20
P,S	**sulfaphenazole**, substc.	mg/dl	0,031 81	mmol/l	31,44	314,36
P,S	**sulfapyrazole**, substc.	mg/dl	0,030 45	mmol/l	32,84	328,39
P,S	**sulfapyridine**, substc.	mg/dl	0,040 11	mmol/l	24,93	249,29
P,S	**sulfathiazole**, substc.	mg/dl	0,039 17	mmol/l	25,53	255,31
P,S	**sulfisomidine**, substc.	mg/dl	0,035 93	mmol/l	27,83	278,33
dU	**testosterone**, ams.	µg	3,467	nmol	0,288 43	288,429

[P] Some laboratories will not report individual sulfonamides by name: in such cases the component name is **sulfonamide** (thus, P—Sulfonamide, substc. = x mmol/l).

See page 48 for explanation

System	Component & quantity	"Old" unit	Factor old→new	"New" unit	Factor new→old	M_r or A_r
P,S	*thyroxin, substc. ["T₄"]	µg/dl µg/l	12,87 1,287	nmol/l nmol/l	0,077 69 0,776 9	776,874
P,S	tocopherol(417), substc.	mg/dl mg/l	24,00 2,400	µmol/l µmol/l	0,041 67 0,416 7	416,685
P,S	transferrin, massc.	mg/dl	0,01	g/l	100	~80 000
P,S	transferrin(Fe binding sites), substc.	µg/dl	0,179 1	µmol/l	5,585	Fe = 55,847
P,S	*triglyceride, substc.	mg/dl g/l	0,011 29 1,129	mmol/l mmol/l	88,54 0,885 4	glycerol trioleate = 885,445
P	triiodothyronine, substc.	ng/dl	0,015 36	nmol/l	65,10	650,976
P,S	**urate, substc.	mg/dl mg/l	59,48 5,948	µmol/l µmol/l	0,016 81 0,168 1	168,112
dU	urate, ams.	mg	0,005 948	mmol	168,1	168,112

System	Component & quantity	"Old" unit	Factor old→new	"New" unit	Factor new→old	M_r or A_r
P,S	**urea,**[q] substc.	mg/dl	0,166 5	**mmol/l**	6,006	60,055 4
		mg/l	0,016 65	**mmol/l**	60,06	
		g/l	16,65	**mmol/l**	0,060 06	
		urea-N, mg/dl	0,357 0	**urea, mmol/l**	2,801	N = 14,006 7
		urea-N, mg/l	0,035 70	**urea, mmol/l**	28,01	
dU	*urea,*[q] ams.	g	16,65	**mmol**	0,060 06	60,055 4
		urea-N, mg	0,035 70	**urea, mmol**	28,01	N = 14,006 7
		urea-N, g	35,70	**urea, mmol**	0,028 01	
dU	**urobilinogen,** ams.	mg	1,687	**µmol**	0,592 7	*i*-urobilinogen = 592,733 8
(B)Erc	**uroporphyrins(I + III),** substc.	µg/dl	12,04	**nmol/l**	0,083 08	830,77
		µg/l	1,204	**nmol/l**	0,830 8	
dU	**uroporphyrins(I + III),** ams.	µg	1,204	**nmol**	0,830 8	830,77
	vanilmandelate *see* 4-hydroxy-3-methoxymandelate					

[q] The recommended name is **carbamide.** This has frequently been reported in terms of urea nitrogen ("BUN", for blood) but it is now recommended that it be reported as urea. Factors are given for converting (*a*) numerical values for urea in mass units into numerical values for urea in substance units and (*b*) numerical values for urea nitrogen in mass units into numerical values for urea in substance units.

See page 48 for explanation

System	Component & quantity	"Old" unit	Factor old→new	"New" unit	Factor new→old	M_r or A_r
	vitamin A *see* retinol					
	vitamin B-12 *see* cyanocobalamin					
	vitamin C *see* ascorbate					
	vitamin E *see* tocopherol					
	VMA *see* 4-hydroxy-3-methoxymandelate					
P,S	Zn: **zinc(II)**, substc.	μg/dl	0,153 0	μ**mol/l**	6,538	65,38
		mg/l	15,30	μ**mol/l**	0,065 38	

See page 48 for explanation

Physiology

Quantity	"Old" unit	Factor old →new	"New" unit
energy; quantity of heat	cal_{th}	4,184	**J**
	$kcal_{th}$	4,184	**kJ**
	$kcal_{th}$	0,004 184	**MJ**
work	kp·m	9,807	**J**
	kgf·m	9,807	**J**
force	kp	9,807	**N**
	kgf	9,807	**N**
power	kp·m/min	0,167	**W**
	kgf·m/min	0,167	**W**
vascular resistance	$dyn·s/cm^5$	0,1	**kPa·s/l**
	mmHg·min/l	8	**kPa·s/l**
resistance to flow (airways)	$cmH_2O·s/l$	0,098 07	**kPa·s/l**
pressure[a]	mmHg	0,133 3	**kPa**
	cmH_2O	0,098 07	**kPa**

[a] For mmHg see tables on pages 38-40 and nomogram on back cover; for cmH_2O see table on page 41.

Radiation

Quantity	"Old" unit	Factor old → new	"New" unit
absorbed dose; absorbed dose index; kerma; specific energy imparted	rad	0,01	**Gy**
absorbed dose rate	rad/s	0,01	**Gy/s**
activity	Ci	$3,7 \times 10^{10}$	**Bq**
		$3,7 \times 10^4$	**MBq**
		37	**GBq**
dose equivalent	rem	10^{-2}	**J/kg**
exposure	R	$2,58 \times 10^{-4}$	**C/kg**
		0,258	**mC/kg**
exposure rate	R/s	$2,58 \times 10^{-4}$	**C/(kg·s)**
		0,258	**mC/(kg·s)**

Miscellaneous ("Old") Units that Should no Longer be Used

"Old" unit (symbol in parentheses)	Factor old ➞ new	"New" unit
ångström (Å)	0,1	**nanometre (nm)**
atomic weight unit (awu); dalton	0,992 1	**unified atomic mass unit (u)**
micron (μ)	1	**micrometre (μm)**
millimicron (mμ)	1	**nanometre (nm)**
svedberg, Svedberg unit (S, Sv)	10^{-13} 0,1 100	**second (s)** **picosecond (ps)** **femtosecond (fs)**
torr (Torr)	0,133 3	**kilopascal (kPa)**
γ [gamma]	1	**microgram (μg)**
λ [lambda]	1	**microlitre (μl)**

Relationship of the SI to other "metric" systems

The "metric" system can be traced back to 1791, in which year a committee of the Académie des Sciences (Paris) adopted, as the unit of length, the metre (defined as one forty-millionth part of the earth's meridian passing through Paris, and redefined by the 1st CGPM in 1889 as the distance between two marks engraved on a special bar of platinum-iridium alloy kept in the BIPM; for the present definition, see Appendix 2).

The search for a universally acceptable system of measurement began in 1862, with the convening of an international committee under the sponsorship of the British Association for the Advancement of Science. In 1863 this Committee recommended a system based on the metre, the gram, and second. In 1873 a similar committee, also sponsored by the British Association, recommended a system based on the centimetre, the gram, and second, which became widely used and was known as the CGS system.

The CGS system, however, did not satisfactorily meet the need for a universal system of units, and the international studies and conferences continued. In 1901 the Italian physicist G. Giorgi proposed a system based on the metre, the kilogram, the second, and an electric unit. Following its endorsement by a number of international organizations, this system also came into widespread use, under the official names "MKS system" or "Giorgi system". The fourth base unit of the system, the ampere, was not finally selected until 1950, after which date the name "MKSA system" was also used. The Conférence générale des Poids et Mesures adopted this system (and added other units to it) in 1954, and renamed it Système international d'Unités (SI) in 1960.

The SI is, therefore, an expanded version of the MKS/MKSA/Giorgi system that has been used since 1901.

Definitions of the SI base units

metre
...the length equal to 1 650 763,73 wavelengths in vacuum of the radiation corresponding to the transition between the levels $2p_{10}$ and $5d_5$ of the krypton-86 atom (11th CGPM, 1960)

kilogram
...the mass of the international prototype of the kilogram (1st CGPM, 1889, and 3rd CGPM, 1901)

second
...the duration of 9 192 631 770 periods of the radiation corresponding to the transition between the two hyperfine levels of the ground state of the cesium-133 atom (13th CGPM, 1967)

ampere
...that constant electric current which, if maintained in two straight parallel conductors of infinite length, of negligible circular cross-section, and placed 1 metre apart in vacuum, would produce between these conductors a force equal to 2×10^{-7} newton per metre of length (9th CGPM, 1948)

kelvin
...the fraction 1/273,16 of the thermodynamic temperature of the triple point of water (13th CGPM, 1967)

candela
...the luminous intensity, in the perpendicular direction, of a surface of 1/600 000 square metre of a black-body at the temperature of freezing platinum under a pressure of 101 325 newtons per square metre (13th CGPM, 1967)

mole
...the amount of substance of a system which contains as many elementary entities as there are atoms in 0,012 kilogram of carbon-12. When the mole is used, the elementary entities must be specified and may be atoms, molecules, ions, electrons, other particles, or specified groups of such particles (14th CGPM, 1971)